AF594276

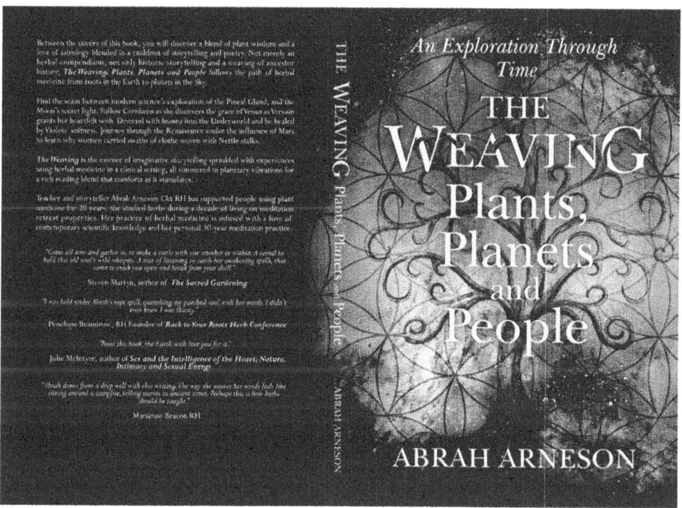
Between the covers of this book, you will discover a blend of plant wisdom and a love of astrology blended in a cauldron of storytelling and poetry. Not merely an herbal compendium, not only historic storytelling and a weaving of ancestor history, The Weaving: Plants, Planets and People follows the path of herbal medicine from roots in the Earth to planets in the Sky.
Find the seam between modern science's exploration of the Pineal Gland, and the Moon's secret light. Follow Ceridwen as she discovers the grace of Venus as Vervain grants her heartfelt wish. Descend with Inanna into the Underworld and be healed by Violets' softness. Journey through the Renaissance under the influence of Mars to learn why women carried swaths of clothe woven with Nettle stalks.
The Weaving is the essence of imaginative storytelling sprinkled with experiences using herbal medicine in a clinical setting, all simmered in planetary vibrations for a rich reading blend that comforts as it stimulates.
Teacher and storyteller Abrah Arneson Clt RH has supported people using plant medicine for 20 years. She studied herbs during a decade of living on meditation retreat properties. Her practice of herbal medicine is infused with a love of contemporary scientific knowledge and her personal 30-year meditation practice.
Steven Martyn, author of The Sacred Gardening
Penelope Beaudrow, RH Founder of Back to Your Roots Herb Conference
Julie McIntyre, author of Sex and the Intelligence of the Heart: Nature, Intimacy and Sexual Energy
Marianne Beacon RH
THE WEAVING Plants, Planets and People
ABRAH ARNESON
An Exploration Through Time
THE WEAVING
Plants, Planets and People
ABRAH ARNESON

THE WEAVING—PLANTS, PLANETS, AND PEOPLE

An Exploration Through Time

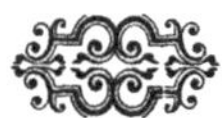

ABRAH ARNESON

Edited by
CHARLENE JONES

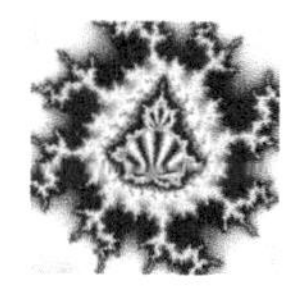

❀ Created with Vellum

Dedication

To women called to practice herbal medicine

CONTENTS

PREFACE

The seed for The Weaving was planted in darkness infused with the rich, moist scent of Earth. In the darkness women sat in a circle on the blankets. In the centre of the circle heat- soaked rocks sparkled with a dusting of dried lavender flowers and sage. From the darkness the women's voices rose speaking of the blessings and the hardships in their lives. After all the words were spoken, the women sang.

The woman who held the space for the circle spoke about Grandmothers. She said, "Your Grandmothers just want you to be happy." And that statement got me thinking.

I asked my Mom about my Grandmothers and Great-Grandmothers. She knew a few stories that were as thin as a worn clothe that no longer keeps you warm. And so I kept thinking.

I checked out a couple of websites that sort through birth, marriage and death certificates. I quickly found out I wasn't looking for dates and names. I wanted to know the stories my Great-Grandmothers told. I wanted to hear the songs they sang. I was really curious about the plants they used for healing and what they grew in their gardens. I wanted to know the simple details of their lives that made them happy.

A little while later, I was at an herbal conference listening to a Cree Elder speak about sacred plants. She asked the predominately White audience to be mindful in using the plants sacred to her community. She explained that without access to these plants her people's culture dies. She used the example of White Sage, a plant used in Indigenous ceremonies that is on the threatened plant list due to loss of habitat and over-harvesting. Without the plant there will be no ceremonies. The songs accompanying the ceremonies will be lost. The reason for the ceremonies will be forgotten. The weaving together of individuals in a community will not take place. She explained that her culture was bound by plants.

And this got me thinking about my culture as a White settler and how we use plants during rituals to create community. Christmas came to mind. There is the Christmas Tree, Mistletoe, Poinsettias, and wreaths of Evergreens. While recalling the moments surrounding these plants bring fond memories to mind, they lack a depth of connection to something greater than my memories of Christmas with my family. The Christmas Tree does not carry a sacred feeling, not like the feeling of White Sage. Most Christmas Trees these days are not even real trees, they are made with PVC plastic. The deep soulful nourishment of the Christmas rituals involving plants is lost. At least it is lost on me. When was the meaning of the Christmas tree lost? When my people crossed the ocean and arrived in a land that looked very different from the naked hills of the Scottish Highlands or England's moors, they lost their plants. With the loss of their plants, they forgot the rituals and stories that accompanied them. I began to wonder not only about who my Great- Grandmothers were, but also how are plants woven into the culture they came from? This question watered the seed for this book.

I began to browse old European Herbals looking for clues and was struck by the rich planetary lore contained in these herbals. Previous to thinking about my Grandmothers and plants, I was aware of the relationship between astrology and European plant medicine but suddenly I had the feeling that the relationship between plants and planets was pointing to a lost language, or a lost way of being in the world, or the thread that if I followed it would lead me to a deeper understanding of who my ancestors were, the stories they told and the events that had shaped their lives.

And so The Weaving began to put down roots and seek the light of day.

There are four major threads that weave this book together. They are stories old as time, plants, planets and people. Let's tease these threads loose and look at each one separately.

The Stories

I have always thought that the best way to learn herbal medicine, with its subtleties and complexities is through story. Have you ever noticed the best herbalists are great storytellers?

Good stories carry advice on how to live in harmony within of the complex web of life. Old stories tell us about the people and the places we come from, what they believed and how they saw the world. Stories that have been passed from one generation to the other, stories that offer medicine are rooted in the nature of the stories in The Weaving.

The stories in this book have shaped me. If you are White and your ancestors settled in a colony somewhere around this planet, these are your stories too. Most of the stories in The Weaving predate the Christianization of Northern Europe, the British Isles and Scandinavia. Some are stories from the Bible, Middle Eastern stories, that Europeans took for their own. And one story in The Weaving has spiralled through time with a message that still shakes the core of any woman living today.

Each story in The Weaving carries the energy of a planet and either has plant medicine as part of it or echoes the medicine found in a plant.

Now just to clarify. Because most stories are a weaving of fact and imagination, and stories change as they spiral through time, I have taken liberty to adjust the shape of some of the stories' details to meet the needs of this time.

Also, because the emphasis of this book is on storytelling, the voice of the book is that of storytellers.

The Planets

I am not astrologer. But I have a deep love of astrology. When I was a little girl on my first day of kindergarten, the teacher ask me as I sat on the braided rug in front of the piano with my new classmates, what song I would like sing, I answered, "The Dawning of the Age of Aquarius." My fascination with astrology started at a young age.

I have also lived with an astrologer for 25 years. Just as he knows a thing or two about herbal medicine from living with me, I have picked up a few things about astrology from him.

Now, that said, this is not a book about medical astrology, although there are references to this system of herbal in The Weaving. Medical astrology involves casting charts of the placement of the planets at the time the illness began to determine the treatment to offer.

In my practice as an herbalist, I do not practice medical astrology. I do however, like to know when and where someone was born and occasionally take a peek at a client's chart, particularly if they are going through a troubling time.

This is also not standard book on astrology. You are not going to find details about what "your Sun" means. Nor will you find predictions about transits and progressions. There is nothing in this book about Moon signs, or for that matter signs like Scorpio, Gemini,

Capricorn and that whole wonderful cast of characters generally found in books about astrology.

In The Weaving the vibration of each planet is explored and how that vibration manifests or does not manifest in the activity of humans, the stories they tell and the plants they use for medicine.

I suspect that my ancestors before there were telescopes that took images of planets creating a sense of a planet's solidity or at least wholeness, experienced the planets as vibrations. Or perhaps the word "forces" is a better choice. They felt the planets as forces in their lives. Sometimes the planets were called Gods.

For example: Renaissance was a dynamic time in the history of Europeans that led to destruction of traditional belief systems and the creation of new ways to experience the world. This creative/destructive force present during the Renaissance mirrors the vibration of Mars. Mars is vibrating with the energy of the polarity between creativity and destruction.

One more thing, I did not explore the outer planets, Uranus, Neptune and Pluto, nor any asteroids, in The Weaving. For this book I was particularly interested in the night sky my ancestors experienced before a telescope spied Uranus in 1781.

The Plants

I am an herbalist. This is how I make my living. I use the medicine made by plants to support the health and well-being of others. My profession is one of the oldest on the planet, probably as old as the professions of Storyteller and Sex Worker.

Being a herbalist is a wonderfully creative and complex profession. I feel blessed to be able to practice herbal medicine. No matter how much I learn, or the amount of experience I gain, there is always more to learn.

Herbal medicine today is enriched by a biomedical model of plant medicine that isolates medicinal constituents from plants and conducts clinical trials. Yet I still find it valuable to travel back in time to try to understand how herbalists who only had their senses to understand a plant's medicine, practiced the art of giving plants to help make a person whole.

Plants are complex beings. They are an intrinsic part of the environment in which they grow. Plants are not only shaped by their environment but they also shape it. Because of their complexity, there are many different ways to talk about plants and the medicine they offer. At one time European herbalists used the vibration of different planets to describe a plant's medicine.

For example: in the 1400s century a herbalist would say, Nettles is ruled by Mars. This statement explained that Nettle like Mars is warm, incites strong feelings, and is both cleansing and renewing.

I find considering a plant's planetary rulership offers a subtle understanding of a plant's medicine. One could call this subtlety the plant's character. For example, plants ruled by the Sun return warmth to a person's heart. I don't mean the physical heart, but the feeling heart, like the expression "warm hands equals warm heart".

Or plants ruled by Jupiter offer the opportunity to

experience the benevolence of life, such as Borage, a plant ruled by Jupiter, and one that brings the courage to the heart.

Understanding the subtle character of a plant's medicine is important in the practice of herbal medicine. For no matter how many plant constituents can be named and sorted through, a plant will be always be more than a sum of its parts. To try to understand a plant's past and how it wove culture together, or not, offers us a more wholistic understanding of its medicine.

Having used herbal medicine long enough to support many, many people, I know a plant's medicine changes more than flesh and bones. It changes the person who takes it. I have found knowing the planetary rulership my ancestors gave to different healing plants helps me understand this less than tangible aspect of herbal medicine.

It is my hope that weaving between the story, the planet and the plant, opens you to a deeper appreciation of a plants' medicine beyond constituents, actions and indications.

One more thing, the plant that is central to each chapter is capitalized out of respect for all it offers to humankind.

People

Since the very beginning, people have gazed upon the stars seeking meaning. Plants have nourished human's bodies, hearts, and minds since before memory. This is how it is. Enough said.

It is my deepest heart wish that these stories, whether you are a White settler or not, make you think about your Grandmothers, their stories, what they saw when they gazed upon the night sky, and the plants that brought them health and joy.

Shall we begin...

PROLOGUE

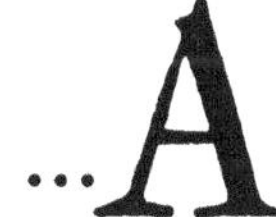nd the Fates fastened the thread of each newborn life to a star. (Dashu. 2017)

THE SUN, CURSES, AND ST. JOHN'S WORT

Imagine you are in a meadow. In the distance you hear the cold North Atlantic drumming against plunging cliffs. You were up at dawn and have walked a long way, through the town, past the farms and beyond the small woods. It is now midmorning. The sun is bright in the sky. It is June 21st, Summer Solstice. You have come to the meadow to gather medicine, medicine that will help you and others when the long nights of winter return.

From a pouch tied to your belt you take out a small clay pot of honey, golden like the rays of the sun. You kneel before a small shrub with bright yellow flowers and pour the honey at the base of its stem and sing:

Behold the joy of children,
Behold the joy of men,
Behold the burning circle
That never has an end. (Eurielle & Ryan Louder, 2017.)

. . .

After pausing for a moment in the morning light, you begin to explore the plant's medicine. Opening to your intuitive sense, you humbly ask the plant to show you its medicine beginning with its yellow flowers.

Golden yellow, the colour of the flowers, is a signature of the Sun. The yellow colour is also associated with the solar plexus, the centre of solar energy in your body. The solar plexus is part of your body's energetic anatomy located in front of the spine and behind the xiphoid process, the smallest region of the sternum. When you are centred in the solar plexus, you walk with confidence in the goodness and strength inherent in your being.

You count the petals on the flowers. They are five, in the shape of a five-pointed star. A Pentagram is a five-pointed star. In ancient medicine circles the Pentagram represented the balance of the elements in health. It is also a symbol of protection against 'evil forces.' The balance of earth, water, fire, air and mind that the Pentagram represents is still believed the best protection against 'evil forces.'

You now know this common flowering weed found in meadows on Midsummer's Eve supports a sense of personal power and brings balance to life.

Next you pick a small sprig of the plant and take a closer look at the leaves. When looked at from above they form a cross. The cross is a common symbol in Christianity, but we are in a meadow on an island off the western coast of Europe, an island that is the land of the Celts. Looking at this simple plant, you ask yourself what the cross meant to the people who lived here before Christianity came to these isles.

The Celts used the symbol of the cross to represent the point where the eternal energies of the self, nature, heaven and earth are bound together. The centre of the cross is the knot that binds matter with spirit.

Lastly you notice the underside of the leaves has small holes. Your botanist self knows these are glands, but intuition suggests these small holes are spaces where the light comes in. As Leonard Cohen sang in his provocative song Anthem, "There is a crack, a crack in everything, that's how the light gets in."(Cohen. 1992). The small holes represent the crack, the tear, the flaw, the rift, that lets the light in.

You pick a flower bud and squeeze it between your fingertips. Rich red-purple oil seeps from the crushed bud like blood from a wound, and the deepest meaning of this plant's medicine is revealed. It heals blood, or more precisely blood lines.

The plant you have chosen to spend time with on this beautiful first day of summer is St John's Wort, a plant ruled by the Sun. In your astrological chart, the Sun represents the place where you shine. It is your light. Your inner Sun creates the gravitational field that pulls those you love close and attracts what you need. Your Sun represents the gifts you have to offer to the world. It is your personal power, your unique potential and truth. The Sun represents your ability to take ownership of who you are and where you came from. It is the most powerful healing planet in your chart.

Astrologers say that if you think you are cursed,

seek the Sun in your chart. A curse is like a shadow cast over your belief in your own goodness, your wholeness, your power to move through the world with kindness and strength. A curse tarnishes your gifts. Your inner Sun shines its lights in these shadowy spaces and chases darkness from mind and heart.

Curses often follow families in the form of depression, addictions, abuse. Family curses have been around for a long time. The Bible lists many. For one, God cursed any man who worshipped any other God.

> You shall not bow down to them or serve them, for I, the Lord your God am a jealous God, visiting the iniquity of the fathers on the children to the third and the fourth generation of those who hate me (Exodus 20:5).

AND THEN THERE IS THE CURSE FOR JUST BEING BORN, the curse of mothers, "Behold, I was brought forth in iniquity, and in sin did my mother conceive me." (Psalm 51:5)

And there is the most famous Biblical curse that many believe brought all the troubles we find in life,

> To Adam he said, "Because you listened to your wife and ate fruit from the tree about which I commanded you, 'You must not eat from it.' Cursed is the ground because of you, through the painful toil you will eat food from it all the days of your life." (Genesis, 3:17)

THE CHRISTIAN GOD IS NOT THE ONLY GOD WHO throws down curses when feeling jealous or when entitlement clouds his judgement.

Dian Cecht, the great healing God of the Celts, was a jealous God who brought extraordinary cures to many. Once he blessed a well with waters that healed soldiers' wounds. The only wounds the waters could not heal were the loss of limbs.

He saved Ireland when Heaven's Queen gave birth to a child so ugly that other gods deemed the child evil. Dian Cecht was asked to kill the infant. Slicing open the infant's heart, he found three serpents. After a fierce battle, the great healer slayed the serpents by throwing them in fire. He spread their ashes in a river. The river boiled and frothed. All life it contained perished. The Celts shuddered with horror to think of what would have happened had the child with such evil in its heart been allowed to live.

On the battlefield the King of the Celts, King Nuada, lost his arm to a sword. Dian Cecht fashioned a silver arm for the King. The King, grateful for Dian Cecht's attention to his wound, honoured him with a celebration. While Dian Cecht was being feted, his son Miach searched the battlefield for the King's severed arm.

When he found the arm, he laid his hands on it and began to sing a healing song:

Joint to joint of it,
And sinew to sinew.

Muscle to muscle of it,
And vessel to vessel.
Strength to strength of it,
And habit to habit. (Dashu. 2017).

MIACH SANG ALL DAY AND ALL NIGHT CAREFULLY weaving life back into flesh and bone. When he was done, the King's silver arm was replaced with one made from flesh. Miach was celebrated as the greatest healer of all time. His fame spread far and wide, reaching his father's ears.

Dian Cecht, hearing whispers that his son's gifts had surpassed his own, flew into a jealous rage. Pretending he wanted to honour his son's accomplishments he called Miach to his home.

Father and son sat down at the kitchen table and to celebrate had a drink. At first Dian Cecht actually thought he might be able to take pleasure in his son's accomplishments. So, he poured them another drink. And another. The drink seeped into the jealousy lurking in Dian Cecht's heart. He began to boast about the many great healings he had performed. Miach was becoming uncomfortable. He could feel the malice behind his father's words and made an excuse to go.

"What? Am I not good enough to drink with?" his father slurred. They had another drink.

Dian Cecht, with a sneer, spoke of the King and his praise for Miach. Jealousy, well-watered, roared from the healer's heart. He smashed his glass on the table, spilling its drink and drew his sword. Without thought

Dian Cecht brought the razor-sharp blade down on his son's head ripping the flesh. Blood flowed. Miach healed the wound with ease.

Blind with rage now, Dian Cecht smashed his sword on his son's skull cracking it open. The sound of the breaking bone was terrible to hear. Miach quickly healed his fractured skull.

The dark demon of murder entered Dian Cecht heart. He raised his sword once more cleaving his son's head in two. Bloody and broken Miach lay dead on the kitchen floor.

A neighbour hearing the shouting and cries coming from Dian Cecht's house ran for Airmed, Dian Cecht's daughter, who was selling eggs at the market in town. Airmed deeply loved her brother. Seeing him on the floor, her father's bloody sword next to the body and the empty bottle on the table she sobbed with sorrow that should never be felt. Her father was nowhere to be seen.

Day passed to night, and Airmed fell into a dark, restless sleep lying on the floor next to her brother's body. When morning Sun broke through the darkness that had settled into her father's house, Airmed carefully gathered up her brother's broken body and carried it to a field out back. Blinded with tears she buried him.

Spent, covered in her brother's blood and the dirt of his grave, she sat down and wept and wept and wept all the terror, all the remorse, all the heartbreak. After three days of weeping, a little chickadee landed on her shoulder and sang its gentle song. She looked up. Sunlight lifted the veil of grief and she saw before her flowers blooming on her brother's grave. From each one of her tears a healing plant had blossomed on her beloved brother's grave.

Airmed took her cloak from her shoulders and laid it upon the Earth. With a prayer in her heart for all those who carry wounds that will not heal, she picked the healing plants and placed them on her cloak.

The oldest tales of Airmen tell that she gathered 365 plants from her brother's grave to place on her cloak—one for each joint and sinew, one for each day of the year, and one for each illness that ever had been or ever would be.

Dian Cecht, shame brewing in his heart, put on the mantle of pride and sought his daughter to make her understand. When he saw her sitting amongst the plants on his son's grave, shining with her new found plant wisdom, he pushed his daughter aside and flung her cloak high into the sky. All the healing plants flew across the sky scattering over meadows and forests, valleys and steep hillsides. In his wrath, he cursed all healers to come. Never again would it be easy to gain the knowledge of plants. One would need to travel far and wide to gather the medicine and knowledge needed to heal.

In very old versions of this story, it is said that Airmed's cloak was the night sky and that each of the healing plants was a star. When Dian Cecht tossed the cloak, the stars fell to earth. Each star became a seed from which a healing plant took root.

While it was Dian Cecht that sent the plants far and

wide, it was Airmed's sorrow, her tears, and prayers that brought us the medicine of the plants.

I remember once complaining to my teacher, "I am so tired of crying," and her response was "when you finish crying, you will be finished". I thought for a long time that this meant that one day my tears would dry up and I would be happy. But life is not that simple, nor easy. Now I understand her words differently. To not be able to cry is to harden like barren soil, cracked in the sun. Tears wash away the sorrow and water the love in the heart making medicine strong. The Sun's light is always clearest after a storm.

Astrologers have another saying, "The Sun's light cannot grow strong without struggle".

Airmed must have known the rage she would incite in her father as she cared for her beloved brother's remains. She must have trembled as she gathered the healing plants from his grave and arranged them on her cloak. She must have watched in horror and terror as her father thundered and roared, scattering the plants across the hills and valleys.

Yet she remained strong in her love for her brother and in her commitment to doing right by him. While the plants were scattered, Airmed kept the knowledge of their healing gifts in her heart and mind despite her father's jealousy and threats. Even today it is said that if you need a plant's medicine call to Airmed and she will guide you. Her spirit remains in the hills and valleys, forest and meadows, wherever healing plants grow.

Airmed must have had a strong inner Sun to withstand the curse her father laid down and remain true to her calling and gift.

I imagine St John's Wort was the plant representing the Sun on Airmed's cloak. St John's Wort carries the light of the Sun. The plant, like morning sunlight, gently opens eyes to see the beauty in one's heart. St John's Wort guides one back to the truth in their heart, the centre of their gravitation field.

St John's Wort carries the medicine of the knot in the centre of life that binds matter with spirit. It is the plant that guides us to our inner Sun, shining brightly. The Sun chases away the shadows that obscure our sense of purpose and opens us to the myriad possibilities present every morning of our lives.

St John's Wort is a popular herb to take for depression. What is depression but the hopelessness that one's life purpose will never be fulfilled? The darkness that arrives with depression is the loss of the one's solar power. St John's Wort is the plant that finds the rip in depression's shadowy shroud and lets the light in.

Like depression, curses: addiction, poverty, health afflictions, and the most stubborn of all, belief systems, tend to run in families. The modern terms for curses are intergenerational trauma, or trans-generational trauma. These curses are repeated in violent words and actions, subtle or outright, and crippling beliefs that cast dark shadows over hearts. These dark shadows are passed from one generation to the next. Simply put, one is destined to relive the pain of one's parents until someone in the family sees deeply into the complex threads of twisted beliefs and unexpressed pain and says, 'No more'. In other words someone finds their inner Sun.

Miach was centred in his inner Sun when he healed the King's arm. He understood his gifts and was able to use them for the benefit of many. He was fearless and determined. It would not have been pleasant sitting for days and nights in a battlefield with a severed arm, healing what is impossible to heal. Miach's Sun shone so brightly, it cast light on what would happen if he did not use his gifts.

When King Nuada lost his arm in battle he also lost his power as king. Celtic Kings were not like today's Royals in gossip magazines. A king in the days of Airmed and Miach were the Earth's consort. The Celtic King, as symbol of the Sun, was responsible for the fertility of the fields, meadows and forest. King Nuada was the human embodiment of the Sun's warmth that brings Earth back to life after a cold, dark winter. The King's purpose was to bestow rebirth. If the King was in any way unwhole, his virility was lost and Earth's abundance would not awaken in the spring. When King Nuada lost his arm, it was not just his position as king at stake, but the life of all the Celts. An unwhole king was a curse upon the land, the farmers, the weavers, the mothers, the children, the cattle, the sheep. Only pestilence, famine, hail and drought would follow such a wound.

When Miach sat down to heal the King's arm, I imagine he took herbal allies with him. I am sure one of those allies was St John's Wort. It is a plant that not only heals wounds of soul such as those rooted in depression but also wounds of the flesh. Remember St John's Wort is the centre point of the cross where spirit and matter are knotted. It heals both matter and spirit.

Once a woman came to me who had raw, weeping, and at times bleeding, eczema on her left calf. The rash ran from her ankle to just below her knee. She had had this rash for 3 years and had tried everything to heal it, but nothing worked. It seemed everything she put on the wound made it worse. She was desperate. The wound was painful and it burned.

St John's Wort, known for healing burns, came to mind. I had her make a paste of St John's Wort infused oil and Slippery Elm bark to plaster over the wound every night. She covered the herbs with a sock to keep the medicine in place while she slept. The wound was completely healed in a month's time with no scarring. I worked with this woman over the next ten years as her family herbalist, during which time the wound never came back.

While knees and calves are represented by Saturn in medical astrology as the manner in which we take a stand, arms and hands of the body are ruled by Mercury, the planet of dexterity. It is significant that the King's arm was cut off.

One could say Mercury handles reality. Mercury shapes the constantly shifting experience of life. But is it the shining of our inner light that determines which reality we will shape, that determines what we give or what we hold back?

These actions of give and take performed by our arms and hands mirror our feelings of personal power, our sense of belonging, and our belief in ourselves. Our point of view, how we look out into the world—that determines the actions of our hands. And we spiral back to the Sun, shining its light into the world, the light both shining on what we choose to believe and revealing what others see.

It is with our hands that we touch life. How we touch life depends upon what we carry in our hearts, whether the warm generosity of the Sun, or a cold, bitter depression that shrouds the Sun's light. How could a king rule benevolently if he was not in touch with his people and the land? How can a family wound be healed if no one is willing to touch it?

The Sun rules the heart. It gets to the heart of the matter. When we live in balance our heart sparks with the creative force that shapes a generous reality. Walking in the light of our inner Sun allows us to give from our eternal heart. It gives us the power to touch any wound, no matter how raw or weeping.

When we live inside a generational trauma, often we do not know how to reach for what will nourish and sustain us. Nor do we know the gifts we carry. Living in community alongside others can be confusing when we do not know how to honour the unique gifts our presence offers. The trauma, or the curse, cripples us. Our open hands become closed fists. There is no inner light, only darkness. Having lost our inner light, we search outside for wholeness, often pulled by the gravitational field of another's Sun just to feel a little warmth.

To heal trauma, find your Sun. How do you find your Sun? Joseph Campbell, a mythologist who outlined the

Hero's Journey (which is a solar myth), advised, "Follow your bliss".

Think of the day you spent in the meadow on the summer solstice, sun-kissed amongst the wildflowers. Remember the joy of singing as you explored the mysteries of St John's Wort. Think of this as a day full of blissful ease. St John's Wort is like a ray of Sun lighting the core of your being where bliss resides.

At home you prepare medicine with the flowers you gathered when the Sun was at its zenith. When dark days return and voices from the past cast shadows over the light you carry in your heart, you take the medicine you made during summer solstice. The ruby-red liquid, slightly bitter to taste, mingles with the light you carry, brightening it once again until you walk in your truth no matter what stories are told. And as the Sun reveals itself, from your hands tumble many gifts.

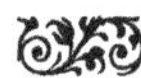

THE SUN, LOST SOULS, AND ANGELICA

The Sun's warmth is generous and full of hope. The Sun beckons us to emerge from shadows, and bloom. The Sun inspires the best in us. Northern people know this. On the first warm spring day, Northerners come out of their houses, turn their faces towards the Sun and smile.

In the north the Sun is a Goddess: gentle, loving and healing. During midsummer rituals when the Sun rides high in the sky, Celts honour Aine, the Goddess of summer, love and wealth. Our bright life-giving star is named after the Norse goddess Sunna, a Goddess known for her kindness. Europe's oldest Sun Goddess belongs to the Sami, the Indigenous people of Scandinavia. She is Beaivi, the Goddess who blesses plants, reindeer and sanity.

The Sami do not anthropomorphize Beaivi. She is not a Goddess with long flowing hair and radiant beauty. Nor is she old and wrinkled. I am not even sure if we can give Beaivi a gender from a Western cultural point of view or even call her a Goddess. Beaivi is the gentle, glowing caress that thaws frozen waters, warms the earth and awakens plants from their deep winter slumber.

One of the first plants to receive Beaivi's blessing and awaken is Angelica. In early spring, while the North and South Winds fight for sovereignty over the frozen Earth, Angelica rises like a flame and calls to the beloved Sun, "I am here." Angelica reaches for the Sun like a lover longing for her beloved's touch. Angelica belongs to the Sun. And like the Sun, Angelica is a generous plant. In early spring when food is still scarce, Angelica nourishes the reindeer who have pushed through deep snows all winter long, and the bear who has just awoken from dream.

How Angelica received its name is a well known story. It was the mid 14th century. The Black Death was sweeping across Europe indiscriminatingly harvesting the souls of the rich, the poor, man, woman and child. Rotting corpses piled up at the edges of towns. People awoke in the morning feeling well and strong and were dead by night fall. Houses were shuttered, businesses closed, children moved from cities to the countryside in the uncertainty of who would be taken next. Those sweating in their beds with boils bursting with puss, restless with delirium, were abandoned by family and left to their end. It was a terrifying time. There was no remedy for the Black Death.

Then a Benedictine monk (sometimes the story replaces the monk with an Italian physician) had a dream. In the dream Archangel Michael (sometimes the angel is Raphael or Gabriel) appeared and showed him the plant to cure the plague. The plant was Angelica. And so, Angelica was named for an angel and its profound healing virtues were endorsed by the church.

Before the plague years, Angelica was just another weed in ditches all over Europe. After the monk's dream Angelica became precious and was coveted as a plant that could protect your body and soul from the grim death the plague offered. If you had a piece of Angelica root in your pocket you were lucky. It could not only save your life, but it could also make you rich.

As Angelica disappeared from wild places, it reappeared in medicinal herb gardens. Laws were passed to protect the cultivated Angelica. If a man was caught in another's Angelica patch, it was lawful to hit him on the head, knock him down and take his clothes.

Two hundred years later English botanist John Gerard wrote in his famous herbal, "Angelica as a singular remedie against poison, and against the plague, and all infections taken by evil and corrupt aire" (Gerard. 1597).

Today's research shows Angelica's volatile oils have significant anti-bacterial and anti-viral actions. It is effective against: Clostridium difficile, Clostridium perfringens, Enterococcus facealis, Eubacterium limosum, Peptostreptococcus anaerobius, and Candida albicans and staphylococcus aureus and Escherichia coli. It is effective against herpes simplex virus type 1 and coxsackievirus B3. These are just a few of the microorganisms Angelica supports the body in overcoming.

Before the angel appeared in the monk's dream and

before the plagues ravished Europe, Angelica was named for the bear. Northern Europeans called the plant Bear Pipe.

Bear is the great herbalist. Bear knows where the medicinal roots grow and how to make use of their medicine. There is a North American plant called Osha, or Bear Root in many Indigenous languages, that grows in the mountains and foothills of the Rocky Mountains. It is similar to European Angelica.

Osha is named after Bear because it is the first plant Bear seeks when he wakes in the spring. After digging up the root, Bear chews it to a pulp and then spits it all over his body. He then rolls around on the ground to work the medicinal juices deep into his coarse fur. This kills off anything that might have made a home on his body while he slept in his nest of shredded wood and dried leaves. Once he is satisfied that he is nice and clean, Bear seeks out female Bear and offers her a piece of Osha root.

It is said if you dream of Bear, you will be able to learn the secrets of plant medicine. Bears are not only great herbalists. Bears, like monks, are also great dreamers.

Bear carries messages between worlds. Old folk-songs from the mountains in Norway sing about bear's dreamtime journey as she snuggly sleeps through the winter's cold. During the first part of winter, Bear slumbers on her left side, sucking her left paw, and dreams of the past gathering wisdom from ancestors to carry into the spring's renewal. On February 2$^{nd.}$, the day the Celt's marks as the Heart of Winter, Bear turns onto her right side and begins the dream of spring. Bear dreams into being the first warm days when she will emerge from her den, cubs in tow, and seek out medicinal roots. Once refreshed and with a full belly, she dreams of playing her flute.

Bear crafts her flute from the stem of the Angelica plant. When Bear sends her breath through the Angelica's long hollow tube a deep, soulful melody ignites and floats through the forest, over the mountains and to the sea. The flute's song beckons the Sun's generous warmth, calling it to return and enliven the ground-loving Bearberry and the great Oak, tiny Black Fly and soaring Eagle, the leaping Salmon and crawling Worm.

The Sami people make flutes from Angelica's stems for healing ceremonies that bring renewal. But for a healing ceremony to take place, there must be a question burning in your heart, a question that can only be answered by traveling to the land of the lost souls. Angelica's flutes know magical songs that guide you to the land of the dead where you will find lost souls. Once found, Angelica's flutes' enchanting music brings the lost ones homes, and your question will be answered.

Let me tell you a story.

Several years ago, I met a man named Ailo Gaup. He was a Sami man, a journalist and a poet. He wore t-shirts with collars and blue jeans with a belt. He had a round belly, a handsome brown face and sparkling blue eyes. He loved to play and laugh. Once when we were picking blackberries on a sunny July day, delighting in the berries' sweet warmth, Ailo threw himself on the ground, rolled onto his back and kicked his feet into the air growling like a bear with a belly full of berries. Ailo was a shaman. He carried Bear's medicine.

There is a healing song Ailo sang. It is a timeless song, a song he learned from a very old woman with wrinkles deep as river canyons. She lived on the northern tip of Greenland and had slept through many dark winters. When Ailo sang the song the old woman taught him, souls came home. The sacred song Ailo sang is called the Bear's Song. Its bittersweet melody rises and falls like a flute's sorrowful call.

The Bear's Song travels far across space and spirals through time. The Bear's Song unburdens the lost souls of the grief that exiles them to forgotten lands. It unravels the hurt that cannot be explained and thaws the horror that has frozen in their eyes. The Bear's Song caresses the heart's longing to be whole. When the song is over, and silence fills all space, the soul is whole, and the heart radiates like the Sun.

Angelica flute's song, like Bear's Song, touches deep longings in the soul and can be bewitching. I wonder if the Pied Pipers' flute was made from an Angelica stem. The Piper understood the magic of songs and flutes. I imagine he was a shaman who carried Bear medicine from the North and traveled the land offering his healing music to those in need. That is how he arrived in Hamelin to help the people rid themselves of rats.

Hamelin was overrun by rats. There were rats everywhere. In the church, in the mill (especially in the mill), in the gardens, in the ale house, in the houses, in the street. There were more rats than people and cats. The townspeople were frightened for they knew rats carried disease. How were the people in Hamelin going to rid themselves of the nasty, filthy rats?

One day a strange looking fellow arrived in the village. His clothing was colourful, much too colourful for the devout people of Hamelin. He wore bells that jingled as he walked. His walk was more like a dance. The stranger was small in stature, but a little plump and had a mischievous twinkle in his eye. The people of Hamelin were wary of the stranger for they did not wear colourful clothes and they certainly did not wear bells. The people of Hamelin hoped he would not stay. He was too strange for the likes of them.

When the Mayor asked the stranger his business, the stranger replied, "I have come to rid your village of the rats." The Mayor laughed and scoffed at the man's appearance, snickered at his funny accent and mimicked the way he walked. The villagers howled and imitated the Mayor's mocking of the stranger.

The stranger added, "For a price, of course," wondering why he was bothering with such people.

The Mayor threw the man in colourful clothing a threatening look, "How dare you come to my village, you foreign charlatan, and make claims of curing the grave misfortune my people suffer."

The stranger answered, "I assure you I am serious about my offer."

The Mayor's wife who was standing next to him, nudged her husband with her elbow. She had heard of the magical powers men like the piper had. "What do you have to lose? If he can do it you are a hero and if he cannot, no one will blame you," she whispered in the Mayor's ear.

The mayor puffed himself up as he prepared to negotiate, "If you rid Hamelin of the rats, what do you want in return?"

The stranger said, "Gold. 1000 gold coins."

The Mayor coughed when he heard the strange man's price and his wife nudged him again and the Mayor agreed, "It's a deal. If you rid our good village of the rats, we will pay your price."

Shaking the Mayor's hand, the stranger promised, "By night fall there will be no rats in this village." And he took his flute from his pocket.

It was an eerie bewitching tune the stranger played on his Angelica flute. Its hypnotizing melody floated through the cobbled streets of Hamelin, around corners and through windows. The tune mesmerized the towns folk, and they stood listening as if frozen in time.

Suddenly a whirling scurrying sound filled the village and a thousand rats burst from every nook and cranny. The rats hurried towards the stranger, enchanted by the music played on his flute. As the stranger walked towards the outskirts of the village, still playing his haunting song, the 1000 rats followed him.

When he arrived at the sea the rats, spellbound by the music, raced into the water. Waves washed over them and pulled them out to sea. All the rats of Hamelin drowned.

When the stranger returned to the town of Hamelin, he expected a hero's welcome. But that was not what the good people of Hamelin offered him. The people, while happy that the rats had left, were fearful of the magic the stranger had woven with his flute. They whispered amongst themselves that he was an enchanter. The Mayor accused the stranger of being in the service of the devil and refused to pay the promised fee.

The stranger, not happy that the people had turned their backs on him and reneged on their part of the bargain, turned to leave the village with a scowl on his face but not before saying, "I will be back in one year. And you will be sorry."

As the year passed, the people of Hamelin forgot bit by bit about the stranger and their broken promise. Then one year later from the very day the rats drowned in the sea, the stranger returned. He walked through the village, his flute playing an eerie tune. The melody wafted through the streets, around corners and into windows of the quiet village of Hamelin. One by one, the children of the village began appearing from behind closed doors, back alleys and surrounding fields dancing to the bewitching music. And when the stranger headed to the outskirts of the village the children followed him. None of the children were ever seen again.

This is a creepy story for a child's bedtime. But aren't most fairy tales creepy? What is chilling about this fairy tale is the truth in it. In 1282 one hundred and thirty children disappeared from Hamelin and no one remembers why. The only record of this troubling loss is a shattered stain glass window in the town's church. There is no record of rats or a piper from 1282.

It was 250 years after the children disappeared that

the rats and the Piper arrived in Hamelin's tragic story and the village became a warning about the plague and a treacherous stranger whose magic was for sale. Around the same time the Pied Piper appeared as the culprit in the missing children of Hamelin, Bear Pipe was renamed Angelica. It was also about this time that monks began to plant Angelica in their gardens to ward off witches, while women planted Angelica to protect them from the witch hunter's evil eye.

The story of the Pied Piper was conjured during the burning times in Germany as traditional healers, herbalists and midwives were hunted down, tied to a stake and set on fire. Some villages during this dark time in history were left with only one woman after the witch hunters rode out of town with pockets full of gold. Gold was the price they charged for saving villages from women in cahoots with the Devil.

The curious thing about this fairy tale is the Pied Piper becomes the villain in the story, while the Mayor who breaks his promise and the townspeople who turn their backs on the stranger are viewed as reasonable. The story tells us it is okay not to honour traditional healing rituals and suggests it is better to live with the trauma we know than the healing we do not, or perhaps put another way, the devil we know rather than the angel we don't. The fearful wariness of the villagers for the unknown the story insinuates, is not the nature of the Sun. Nor is it the nature of Angelica.

The Sun shines and brings warmth to all of life. It does not hold back its gifts for only the chosen few.

Angelica, a plant that grows in ditches, offers medicine to all. This is the way of the Sun.

Try to image what it was like in the mid 1500's when the Piper and his flute became part of the horrible story of Hamelin's lost children. The plague two hundred years earlier had killed entire families in a single day. A shoemaker from Tuscany wrote:

> Father abandoned child, wife husband, one brother another; for this illness seemed to strike through the breath and sight. And so they died. And none could be found to bury the dead for money or friendship. Members of a household brought their dead to a ditch as best they could, without priest, without divine offices. (Gerard. 1597).

The plague ravished Europe in the mid 1300's. By the 1500's the infectious disease continued to rise up as if from nowhere and carry away children and the elderly, but it was not as lethal as it had been two centuries earlier. The ongoing fear of sickness and death, the horrors experienced just a few generations earlier, must have left a hollow emptiness, a darkness, a terror, in Europe's soul.

Three hundred years later Europe was again ravished by death. Fields were soaked in blood and mass burials carried out on the edges of towns. Twenty million died on European soil during World War 1.

It is unsettling that both the plague and World War I took 20 million European lives. Even more disturbing, it seems that part of the mourning rituals included the murder of innocents. Someone had to be blamed for all the death and suffering. The plague was one justification for the deaths of at least 80,000 women during the Burning Times. The trauma left behind by WWI is directly linked to the horrors of Holocaust. The murder of both women and Jews followed a time of intense trauma.

As corpses were disposed of in mass graves, both during the witch hunts and later the holocaust, it was said that the persecuted were the ones who brought the terrible suffering down on ordinary people. There was an unyielding belief that the one who was different needed to be destroyed to ensure everyday people could live in peace and harmony. Is this what happens when ancient healing traditions are disrespected, demonized and lost?

If there was ever a time when Angelica's medicine is needed, it is following mass trauma.

Herbalists say Angelica's hollow stem understands the medicine needed to heal the hollowness left behind by trauma. They say Angelica is for the person who has become hollow. A hollow person has lost their will. They feel no purpose. It is like a howling wind has ripped through the very core of their being and blown out the spark of fire carried in the heart, the spark that is a gift from the Sun. When someone is hollow, their heart becomes cold. When a heart is cold, the soul is lost. The light of their inner Sun is extinguished.

I remember when a hollow woman came to the

clinic for help. The skin on her cold hands had a blue twinge. Her hair was limp and dull. Her body, long and thin, sat rigid in the soft cushions of the chair. Her eyes wide with fear scanned the room. She opened her pale lips to speak, and no words came out.

"How can I help?" I asked.

She whispered, "I do not know. I feel hollow."

She was a woman who had barely survived her childhood. Her soul was torn to pieces like one would tear rags from an old sheet. She no longer knew how to ask for help. She no longer knew what she needed. She no longer had words of her own.

I offered her Angelica hoping its warmth would ignite a small flame in heart, warming her once again. Angelica medicine carries the gentle warmth of springtime's Sun, the warmth that calls to the frozen longing for life hidden deep inside winter's darkness. Angelica like the Sun knows how to awaken springtime's seeds of hope, creativity and joy. Angelica infused with Sunshine contains the sparks that lights the way home for lost souls.

After a few months of tender encouragement, patient listening and daily doses of Angelica she dropped by the clinic unexpectedly. This was a good sign I thought.

Spontaneity is a kind of generosity that allows life to unfold, uncontrived like a child's summer day.

She asked me to feel her hands. They were warm. She giggled and said, "Warm hands, warm heart." And gave me a bear of a hug. She told me she was beginning to remember who she was.

ABRAH ARNESON

THE MOON, FALLING IN HOLES, AND MUGWORT

During the first days of May, Mugwort, a plant ruled by the Moon, appears inconveniently in the garden where Calendula, a plant beloved by the Sun, grows. Mugwort's shoots emerge from the damp garden soil and into the light of spring, twisting like snakes waking after a long winter of dreams.

A common wayside weed, Mugwort is not particularly welcome in gardens. Herbalists prefer Mugwort to grow wild along fence lines or at the edge of an undomesticated field where the trees begin to grow taller and forests start to take shape.

Mugwort really could care less about what gardeners or herbalists want. This wily plant will seed itself into the most domestic, carefully manicured places and, like threads of a disturbing dream weaving itself into morning's light, Mugwort never quite goes away once it has made itself known.

Mugwort is a dreamer's plant. It is a friend to those who like to explore beyond fence lines, wayside places and edges of forests. It is an oneiric, a plant that cultivates dreams. As I prepare to write about Mugwort, I ask Mugwort to appear in a dream and teach me what I can learn.

For many years I have watched my dreams and the dreams of others, trying to tease out the meaning of peculiar nighttime wanderings. Often, when a question I cannot answer is pressed upon me I ask for a dream to shine its unearthly light and guide me onto a new path of understanding. Some people call this 'dream incubation'.

The first thing I do to incubate a dream is clarify my question or concern and write it down. For example, if I am concerned about a client, I may write down a question about her underlying health challenge or perhaps ask for guidance on what herbs to use.

Before bed, I politely and with humility ask for a dream and repeat the question three times silently to myself. Then I take 30 drops of Mugwort tincture. As I lie in bed waiting for sleep to arrive, I try to open myself up to the client and sense how her body feels as illness winds itself through her flesh and mind. I imagine placing different herbs over her body and try to become aware of the subtle shifts in energy the plants create in my body feeling her body. Then I sleep and dream.

In the morning when I wake, I ask, "Where was I?" and let the scattered dream images emerge. Once the images have gathered together, I feel them in my body. Lastly, I write them down in my dream journal. I do this for three nights as I seek clarity.

On the first night I asked for a dream about Mugwort's medicine, I dreamt I poured Feverfew flowers into a great crevice in a mountain.

Feverfew, besides being a traditional plant used to control fever, is a plant known to ease migraine pain. More recent research shows it as an antimicrobial plant that crosses the blood-brain barrier. It also contains some anti-cancer properties.

On the second night I dreamt of Wild Ginger creeping through the garden. Wild Ginger is a shy plant with an exotically seductive flower. It prefers to grow next to rotting logs. Wild Ginger warms up cold bodies and minds. It was once called Snake Root.

On the third night I found myself standing in a church next to a baptismal font. This is the place in a church where brides take deep breaths before walking down the aisle, mourners adjust their clothing and pull themselves together, and newborns are hushed before their baptism.

As I pulled open the heavy door to the inner church a figure greeted me. His face and body were painted with orange, white and black stripes. The few clothes he wore were orange and black. His wild black hair was adorned with feathers. Feathers stuck out from strips of cloth tied around his arms, wrists and ankles. He was untamed.

He danced. It was a rhythmic, undulating dance. He circled me, singing in a low guttural voice. As he danced light began to fill my body. Green light. When he stopped dancing, I began. Fluid waves of light flowed from my spinning body as I made my way towards the altar.

I know this is Mugwort's dream and I wake up.

Sitting up in bed, my dog Lily on the floor beside me snoring, I see the sheets crumpled where Mark has been, and laundry sitting folded on the dresser ready for me to put away. I think, how can this be real?

Dreams challenge everyday timelines and distort consensual meaning when allowed to linger in morning's light.

Stories can be like that too. Like dreams, stories can alter everything we thought we knew.

For some, stories about girls falling in holes alter everything. Like the story told by the old Ukrainian woman wearing a red kerchief over her grey hair, neatly tied under the chin as she hangs Mugwort to dry. This story goes like this...

A long time ago, a young girl went into Starodubsk, an old Oak forest, searching for mushrooms to fill her basket. As she wandered, a strange looking root caught her attention. Curious, she crept closer to the root and as she bent to get a better look, she saw the strange root was a nest of snakes. Horrified, she stepped backwards and fell into a hole. It was the hole where the snakes lived.

It was dark in the hole and hissing sounds filled the dank air. Around her ankles the girl could feel the snakes slither as their forked tongues tasted her skin. The girl froze in terror. Just as she was about to collapse in a faint, from deep inside the darkness of the hole a shimmering glow appeared. As the glow brightened and came nearer, the girl could see it was an undulating light, like the light of a full Moon on a still lake. The glow was the golden-horned Queen of Snakes.

The Queen of the Snakes comforted the girl and led her and the snakes to a luminous stone in the centre of the hole. The snakes licked the stone, and their hunger was satisfied. Seeing this, the girl licked the stone as well and her fear disappeared.

For the long, cold winter, the girl, under the protection of the Queen, lived as the snakes lived deep down in the dark hole with the luminous stone that fed and satisfied them all.

When the days grew longer and the earth began to warm, the snakes prepared to return to the surface of the world. Knowing the girl would need their help to climb from the hole, the snakes interlaced their bodies forming a ladder for her.

As the girl said her goodbyes and turned to climb the ladder, the Queen of the Snakes blessed her with the gift of understanding the language of plants. Knowing the plants' language empowered the girl with the gift of plant medicine.

"However," The Queen warned, "Never speak the name Chernobyl or you will lose the gift forever." Chernobyl by another name is Mugwort. In Ukrainian Chernobyl means 'the dark one'.

The girl carried her gift from the Queen of the Snakes for a very long time. She cared for the plants. The plants in turn cared for her. She healed many people and her fame as an herbalist spread far and wide until one day as she walked along a footpath a man asked her, "What is the name of this plant?"

"Oh," she said, "Chernobyl." And her gift vanished.

Old Ukrainian women say this is how Mugwort acquired its other name, Zabytko, "herb of forgetfulness." Forgetfulness is a kind of hole memory slides into.

Have you ever noticed that there are many stories of girls falling down holes?

There is the Germanic story of Frau Holle who welcomes into her cottage an obedient, pretty girl after she falls down a well. After the obedient girl cleans Frau Holle's house and cooks her food, Frau Holle blesses the obedient girl with gold. When a lazy and ugly girl falls into the same well and is not as quick to please Frau Holle as the obedient girl, Frau Holle curses her by pouring sticky black tar over her head.

Alice in Wonderland follows a rabbit down a hole and has many bewildering adventures. Alice's bizarre journey comes to an end when the Queen of Hearts, in a blind fury, throws all her cards at Alice and the girl startles awake.

One of the most famous falls is that of Persephone. Persephone, a Goddess in Waiting, the daughter of Demeter, the great Greek Goddess of the Grain, was sweet with beauty and tenderness. When Hades, the God of the Underworld, caught a glimpse of Persephone's innocence, he had to have her.

Hades confided his desire to Zeus who was an expert at snatching young women. Together they planned Persephone's abduction to the Underworld, the realm of Hades.

There are two versions of this story. In one, Hades and Zeus cause a huge chasm to open in the Earth into which Persephone falls. In another, she is seduced by the sweet scent of flowering Narcissus. When she pulls the flower from the ground, a hole is left behind that begins to grow bigger and bigger. Wide-eyed in horror, Persephone freezes as the Earth thunders with the galloping hooves of Hades' chariot rising from the Underworld. Persephone screams and into the hole she falls. Or was she dragged?

Persephone, like our herbalist in a hole with snakes, does something the Celts say one should never do if you find yourself falling into a hole—never, ever eat any food or drink any drink. It is said if you do you will spend the rest of your life in the otherworld of the hole.

Persephone eats 6 blood red pomegranate seeds while down in Hades. It is only through her mother's stubborn refusal to accept her daughter's fate of living the rest of her life in the Underworld that a deal was struck. The deal Demeter, Persephone's mother, makes is her daughter will be by her side on the sunny side of the Earth for six months of the year. The other six months, Persephone is destined to be the Queen of the Underworld. As Queen of the Underworld, Persephone is feared and shunned as Winter. During the six months above ground Persephone is welcomed as Spring.

There are creation stories from all over the world that tell of a woman falling through a hole in the sky and seeding life on Earth.

Mugwort's family name, Artemisia, comes from one such Goddess, Artemis of Ephesus. In a flash of brilliance Artemis tumbled to Earth bringing with her—life. Today, astrophysicists hypothesize she was a meteor, a rock from Jupiter, that blazed across the sky crashing to earth. In either case, to the ancient ones Artemis was a Goddess who fell through a hole in the sky.

Artemis of Ephesus was the sacred Goddess of the Amazons, a matriarchal society that thrived across North Africa around the same time as the ancient Greeks told Persephone's story.

Amazonian women were the first to wear pants, ride horses and go into battle alongside men. They did not cut off their left breast to be better archers. That is a Greek myth. The Amazonian women were the Greeks' enemies. The women who turned to Artemis for guidance tattooed significant passages on their skin, smoked cannabis and loved bonfires. They had sex with partners of their choice. In their culture parenting was a community responsibility.

In Turkey there is a copy of a wooden statue of Artemis of Ephesus from the 1st century AD with arms opening wide, offering an embrace. Her skirt is carved with animals. Her many breasts are full with boundless nourishment. Artemis' necklace is a swirl of the signs of the zodiac and a snake entwines her hair.

Artemis of Ephesus predates the Greek Goddess Artemisia. The Greeks called their Artemis the Goddess of the Woods. Their stories tell of a stubborn, irrational woman who refused to be seduced by a man.

Artemis of Ephesus however was not opposed to sex. She did however prefer it to be consensual and encouraged women to retain their personal power even in intimate relationships.

The Amazons, under Artemis' guidance, initiated girls at menarche by sending them into the forest to learn to dance like a bear. A girl could not lie with a man until she embodied the power of a bear.

The interesting thing about these girls falling into holes is some returned with superpowers, like our dear Ukrainian herbalist or Persephone or the pretty, obedient girl. Others were shamed like the lazy girl. Some were dismissed as silly girls telling fanciful tales like Alice. Most girls and women who fall down holes become stories barely remembered until they are forgotten. Why is this so?

Let's think about falling in a hole. Holes are dark. There is no external light. Being in a hole is like being enclosed in a very long night. On long dark nights things unseen prowl and slither. Things are done in the dark and tucked away into shadows never to be seen by the light of day. Crimes take place in the dark. Thieves take their bounty in the dark. Witches dance in the dark. Magic happens in the dark. Dreams arrive in the dark.

When life becomes dark, good friends tell us, "Morning always comes." But that is not the case for all girls who fall into holes. Some are trapped. These girls must find the light that arrives before morning or they will continue on in the dark, befuddled and confused, pulled this way or that way, depending on the desire ripening in the shadows.

You may be thinking that the Moon lights up night's darkness. But Moon's light is unreliable. It comes and goes as time passes. If a girl falls in a hole during the dark Moon, there is no Moonlight to guide her.

There is another light in the night, a light we barely notice. It is a light we rarely remember. During the long dark night, there is always dream light.

The dream light unveils worlds never imagined. Dream light illuminates spiralling staircases descending deep beneath ancient fortresses made from stones. Dream light shines on cliffs and falls into an endless blue sky. In dream light wallets are lost and jewels are found. From dream light shadows step, enchanting dark lovers. Or we have tea with the long dead. In dream light flowers talk and anyone can grow cat whiskers and lounge on tree branches watching butterflies or run with coyotes yipping and yapping. Anything is possible in dream light like learning the medicine of every plant ever known from the Queen of Snakes.

Where does the wise light in dreams comes from? No one really knows.

Some biologists, however, are beginning to wonder if dreams, or dream light shines from the pineal gland. About the size of a grain of rice, the pineal gland sits in the middle of your brain slightly to the left.

In the ancient healing tradition called Qigong, this area of the brain is called the Crystal Place.

Qigong Masters teach that within the Crystal Palace there is a Moon. They say the light from this inner

Moon guides us when darkness overcomes our journey. Many theorize that the pineal gland is the inner Moon.

Inside the pineal gland are micro-crystals made from the stone Calcite. Calcite creates the glow on stalactites and stalagmites deep inside caves. Calcite shimmers the rainbow sheen on mother of pearl and offers pearls their soft white glow. Calcite, pearls and mother of pearl are all ruled by the Moon.

Scientists Simon Baconnier, Sidney.B. Lang, and René de Seze describe the potential of Calcite's actions within the pineal gland, "These crystals could be responsible for an electromechanical biological transduction mechanism in the pineal gland due to their structure and piezoelectric properties." (S. Baconnier, S.B. Lang, Rene de Seze. 2002.). Translated into common language: when there is friction or pressure within the pineal an electrical charge is created by the calcite crystals creating light. Think of Moonlight on a bitter cold January night weaving through the trees of a forest, casting dark blue shadows and you will have a sense of calcite's glow.

Judy Hall in The Crystal Bible describes the attribute of calcite this way,

> Calcite is a powerful amplifier and cleanser of energy. Simply having Calcite in the room cleans negative energies from the environment and heightens your energy. Within the body, it removes stagnant energy. The spectrum of colours cleans the physical and subtle bodies. Calcite is an active crystal speeding up development and growth. This is a spiritual stone

> linked to the higher consciousness that facilitates the opening of higher awareness and psychic abilities, channelling, and out of body experiences. It accelerates spiritual development and allows the soul to remember experiences with it returns to the body. (Hall. 2003).

THE PINEAL GLAND SECRETES HORMONES TUNED TO darkness. One of the hormones is melatonin. Melatonin brings healing sleep. It is a powerful antioxidant, inhibits H-pylori, bacteria that cause heart burn and digestive upset, and eases the symptoms of Seasonal Affective Disorder. Taking a supplement of melatonin often enhances dreams—both healing and disturbing.

Another hormone the pineal gland releases is Dimethyltryptamine, commonly referred to as DMT. This is not a very well understood hormone. It is about as well understood as girls who fall into holes, or how the Moon affects plants and the human psyche.

Some people call this hormone "The God Chemical" or the "Big Bang" because it shows up in a big way at the four major portals in life—labour and birth, orgasm and death. These are all times when stories are told about "seeing the light." New life growing in a woman's womb is gently infused with DMT, suggesting life forms in the light of dreams. Small amounts of DMT are also released each night as we enter sleep's darkness.

Let's return to our brave Ukrainian herbalist and take a closer look at her story.

She is in the forest looking for mushrooms. Now we all know in the old days the forest was the place where wolves hunted little girls, or perhaps witches laid traps to eat wayward children. What is our girl doing in the forest by herself? This we do not know. What we know is she is vulnerable, innocent and curious.

She is collecting mushrooms. What kind of mushrooms we need to wonder?

Psilocybin, a favoured magical mushroom used to access alternative perceptions of reality, triggers the release of DMT from the pineal gland. In traditional medicine circles around the world, mushrooms like Psilocybin are used to guide you on healing journeys to rediscover lost wisdom and disconnect from imposed belief systems that limit your life experience. These journeys to other realities are like dreams only more vivid. The journeys can take you deep into the great web of life to experience directly the threads that bind people to animals, to plants, to water, clouds, Sun, Moon, all of life. There are over 200 different types mushrooms known to trigger the release of DMT in the pineal gland and offer the healing experience of life's great weaving.

Had our gentle herbalist heard stories of mysterious mushrooms around the evening's fire? Was she feeling curious about the wonders bestowed upon those who nibbled on mushrooms? Had she taken a tiny bite of a mushroom just before the stick turned into a snake? I wonder if her pineal gland activated, opening her to alternative realities that offer gifts to the brave of heart.

Our herbalist watches the branch turn into a snake

and down the hole she falls. For me, the thought of being in a dark hole, hungry snakes hissing around my feet is to say the least terrifying. Magic, a shift in perception, often happens during intensely stressful moments. This is when the life transforming magic happened for our herbalist. A 'shimmering glow' appeared, like Moonlight softening darkness as it appears from behind clouds or like tinkling calcite crystals turning on the Moonlight that shines from within.

After licking a mysterious stone, luminous like a pearl, our herbalist's fear dissolves along with hunger and she lives with confidence among the snakes and learns their ways. She trusts her inner Moonlight.

And so, she spends the winter in a den of snakes. When spring returns, like Persephone's ascent from the underworld, our herbalist climbs into spring time's glorious soft light. But not before receiving a gift, and what a magnificent gift—the sacred language of plants.

In some cultures, becoming an herbalist is a path of initiation. This is an entirely different form of education from academic learning. Our wise herbalist's journey into the snake's den was an initiation that not only awakened her inner Moon but also taught her how to understand the language of dreams and plants. The snakes, guardians of the medicine of transformation, initiated our herbalist into the healing arts.

Snakes with their unblinking eyes and shedding skins have long been considered great masters of plant medicine. Ancient healers and dreamers from the Asclepius tradition in Ancient Greece sought dreams of snakes to guide them in the use of healing plants to cure diseases of the body, mind and soul. Remnants of Asclepius' wise snakes are still seen in winged double-snake caduceus used as an emblem of doctors and pharmacists today.

Some traditions believe that it is only after one dreams of a plant and its medicine that one is qualified to practice herbal medicine. The dream initiates you into a deeper understanding of a plant's medicine beyond its phyto-constituents and into its place in the great web of life.

Initiation is a very different type of teaching than academic learning. Academic learning is not necessarily focused on direct understanding. It is possible in academic circles to know all the current scientific studies of a plant and have never seen the plant in the wild or even in a garden. Academic learning comes from books and people, not from plants.

Initiation is different. It is secret. The knowledge of initiation is closely guarded. It is only offered when asked. Often the asking for knowledge needs to be done in a particular manner. Sometimes the seeker of knowledge must make an offering and ask several times before the steps to gaining knowledge are offered. In initiation, knowledge does not come from outside oneself but comes from within. It arrives when the inner Moon shines and one connects with the web of life. In plant medicine, knowledge comes from understanding the language of plants, a language without words.

Everything changes with initiation while everything remains the same. Initiation is not for cream puffs or those in a hurry. It is for the brave of heart, recklessly curious and as a last resort. Initiation arrives when that niggle in your heart that says there's more to plant medicine than words in books, or for that matter, more to life than you have been told, grows into a desperate longing for connection. Initiation can be dangerous and demands respect. For this reason, it remains secret.

Following initiation, you know the medicine you carry arrived through hardship. You know your medicine is a gift, a cherished guest carried in your heart. It is not something to boast about or wear as a persona. After initiation, medicine is alive, shining in the inner glow of dreams. Medicine needs to be nourished, cared for, loved, kept sacred, or it is lost.

And as our young herbalist climbs from the snakes' den, she is given a caveat. "You must not tell the name of the 'Dark One'". The Dark One is our humble wayside weed, Mugwort.

The underside of Mugwort's leaves carry the signature of the Moon. They are a soft, gentle white, like Moonlight. Mugwort does not flash the soft, white underside of her lush green growth to any passerby. You must touch Mugwort's leaves and gently turn them over to see their Moon medicine.

Mugwort is the dreamer's herb. According to the online site, *The World of Lucid Dreaming* Mugwort has been used for over 1300 years in rituals to guide one in dreaming.

Those who use Mugwort for dreaming say:

> If you cannot recall your dreams, Mugwort will enhance your dream recall.

> If you dream in black and white, Mugwort will bring colour to your dreams.
>
> If you do not understand language in your dreams, Mugwort will create understanding.
>
> If you cannot steer your dreams, Mugwort will put you in the driver's seat.
>
> If you can steer your dreams, Mugwort will make anything possible. (LaBerge, Ph. D. and Rheingold. 1991)

MUGWORT HAS AN EARTHY SCENT CREATED BY sesquiterpenes. Sesquiterpenes are called phytoconstituents and some speculate it is these that act on the pineal gland. These musty, dank smelling chemicals trigger the cascade of hormones leading to the release of melatonin and DMT activating the calcite crystals' light deep inside the brain.

I prefer to think of Mugwort's affinity to dreams as something we will never be able to name with words, just as initiation can never be explained to the uninitiated and a plant's medicine transcends its individual chemical. Or how stories of herbalists in snake dens awakens our imagination.

It is springtime, the time of renewal, and our herbalist climbs out of the hole, at peace with her inner Moonlight. She knows all the medicine of all the plants, and she carries with her a warning not to be careless with this knowledge.

For several years she journeys through life as an

herbalist sharing her healing gifts from the snakes. One day she tells a man the name of The Dark One, the gift leaves her, and Mugwort takes on the name, Zabytko, "Herb of Forgetfulness."

This to me is even more frightening than a snake pit. Forgetting all herbal knowledge, losing my connection to plants and all the people I know through plants would be devastating. How could our herbalist be so careless? We need to try to understand what happened on the path the day our herbalist lost her medicine.

Let's return to a time when Sun did not mark time. It was Moon and night sky humans turned to for guidance when choosing the right time to hunt and gather, plant and harvest, make medicine and give medicine, make babies and marriage.

At this time all over the world there was worshipped a Great Tree. Different people gave the Great Tree different names. Mayans called it Yaxche. Jewish peoples called it Etz Chaim. Anishinaabe call it Nookomis Giizhig. We are going to visit Northern Europe's Great Tree, Yggdrasil.

A very long time ago, people living where the snow was deep and wolves howled on long winter nights did not see the Milky Way sweeping across the night sky. They gazed upon an ancient tree swaying in the wind. Some called night's starry arch the "Wind Swept Tree" and the sky "the Wide Hand-Basin of the Winds" (Wynn. 2020).

The Norse, Northern Europeans, called this tree Yggdrasil.

There are many stories about Yggdrasil. As with all

old stories spiralling through time, they are fiddled with. Some parts are added. Some parts are omitted. Stories shift and change shape to suit the politics and temperament of the storyteller and the King. This happened to Yggdrasil stories.

Yggdrasil's story is like a dream one can only recall in bits and pieces, hints of meaning here and there, fragments. Yggdrasil's story, at one time a vast tale, can now only bring glimpses into our Northern European ancestor's insight into birth, life, death, ancestors, giants, healing, war, and sacrifice. The fragment of Yggdrasil's story we will unravel is of wise women, the Moon, a well, and snakes.

Yggdrasil's upper branches reach high into heavens, beyond ordinary sight. They are covered in clouds. Yggdrasil's roots burrow deep in the Underworld. There is a well where the roots emerge from the tree's mighty trunk. The well is described as, "a reservoir of ancient Being, fed by a living spring. Its surface ripples and rolls from power and consciousness. Within it resides 'the unfathomable secret of the beginning of life, deeply hidde.'"(Dashu. 2017)

Every night Three Sisters called the Fates leave the Hall of the Moon (the area of the sky the Moon is roaming) and sit by the well. The youngest is Verdani (Becoming), the middle one is called Skuld (Shall be) and the eldest is Urd (Became). The well is named after Urd. It is called Urdrbrunni

Some people call the Three Sisters the Weavers, for every night they sit by the well, twisting, braiding, knotting the threads of Fate. The sisters weave the delicate, complex, unfathomable web of life that contains all life, not only on this beloved blue planet, but across the universe.

When the Sisters are not weaving, they are pouring water from the well over the starry tree's roots. The healing waters trickle over the Great Tree's roots offering a balm to any rot that may weaken their sturdy stance in the Underworld. This is important, for if rot spreads and the roots decay, Yggdrasil will fall and all life will end.

Why do the roots need healing every night? A great snake lives entwined within the roots. The snake is consumed with hunger and seeking satisfaction gnaws on Yggdrasil's roots. Its hunger causes gashes, splits and tears in the roots threatening chaos. This is the chaos that makes human hearts quiver with fear and the dark questions emerge from the shadows of uncertainty, "Is the end near?"

The water the Fates pour over the roots offers the blessings of life. It is said that all the water touches becomes holy. The water is translucent white, like the inner membrane of an egg, the skin over the eye of a snake after it has been shed, or a pearl's glow. Some of this holy water falls to Earth as morning's dew. The old ones called this falling nectar sprinkled over the Earth at sunrise 'honeydew'. They teach it is a nourishing, healing drink that will never diminish.

To me the waters of Urd sound like the light of the full Moon. It is said bathing naked in Moonlight will cure all that harms, both disease and curses as the

Three Sisters, the great weavers of Fate, bless you with the Moon's sweet nectar.

This story was told in a time when people gathered to dance in the full Moon's light, naked. They danced to celebrate life and honour the loving glow of the Moon, no different than the glow of their own inner Moon. They danced to heal, to bless, to conceive, to grieve. They danced the many threads of life the Sisters endlessly weave. They danced in the light hidden to those who only see the light shining on the outside of their skin. Most of the dancers were like our herbalist, women.

Sometime along the way, dancing in Moonlight became sinful, nakedness shameful and Moonlight lost its healing glow. The Moon became the light of madness, depravity and wayward women. It was probably around the same time that our Ukrainian girl herbalist told the man the name of the wayside weed and forgot her medicine.

There is a contemporary herbalist who tells this story and at the end says, "Mugwort is called the herb of forgetfulness because sometimes it is helpful to forget." But I do not believe this is true. When we forget our dreams something inside us dies. When we forget our path, our joy, the hunger for remembrance lies like a snake twisting in our roots gnawing at our sense of belonging. When we forget our medicine, we forget the hardships and wisdom initiation brings. When we forget who we are, we are lost.

Offering a dance in the moonlight to the Three

Sisters is asking for gifts only they can give—the gift of remembering, the gift of knowing and the gift of prophesy. To dance in the Moonlight is a metaphor for dreaming. To know the secret language of dreams is to fall into Urd's well and journey in Moonlight down Yggdrasil's roots plunging deep into the Underworld of initiation or to soar high into its branches and be greeted by ancestors. Mugwort shines the light on your inner Moon dance. Sip a cup of Mugwort tea before bed and slowly over time you will become as wise as the Moon shining in the night.

THE MOON, BLOOD, AND VITEX

I am in a massive ballroom in a downtown hotel. Three grey walls and one of windows overlook an equally grey November city scape. I am sitting at one of many identical round tables, draped with white tablecloths. At each table women of all ages, shapes, colours, and beliefs sip water and politely introduce themselves to each other. This is a conference on woman's spirituality sponsored by Catholic Nuns. It is about to begin.

Like burbles from a large fermentation vat, women's voices bubble up throughout the stale atmosphere of the room as the opening speakers gather on the stage. After the speakers are settled, a big-boned woman takes the microphone.

"Women," her voice booms, silencing the room. She pulls a tampon from her purse. There is nervous laughter. With a theatrical flourish, she removes the tampon from its paper wrapper. There is more nervous laughter. Holding the tampon by its string, she whirls it like a lasso over her head and shouts into the microphone, "WOMEN UNPLUGGED!" and lets it fly.

On cue, drummers begin drumming and the room explodes with joy as hundreds of women leap to their feet and dance. The air sparkles with laughter and gyrating hips flow everywhere.

Women dance. Dancing feels good. Women dance to celebrate life's many moments. Five-year-old girls happily twirl down the street for no reason at all. Teenagers twisting and shaking awaken sexual juiciness. Angry women dance with stomping feet while mourning, women sway wrapped in another's arms.

Women dance around bonfires, in kitchens, in bedrooms, in front of the mirror. They dance on beaches, in forests and in the street on warm summer nights. Women have danced on the hills of Glastonbury, Somerset, England for a very long time.

Glastonbury to the ordinary eye looks like any traditional farming community in Southwest England. Tractors haul hay along the narrow roads. Sheep graze, enclosed in wire fences. In the oldest parts of the town streets and narrow lanes are lined with stone houses. Glastonbury is like most towns throughout the UK.

But if you climb the hills Southeast of Glastonbury, and sit for a minute, calm your mind and gaze upon the valley's curves and hills' rise, off in the distance a veil lifts and you see a woman lying across the land, birthing.

Since women first gathered to dance on the hills cradling Glastonbury, it has been known as sacred lands of the Birthing-Goddess. The landscape unfolds like a woman in voluptuous abandonment, labouring to bring her daughter into the world of men.

Her legs splay across villages and valleys. Her nascent belly is adorned with swaying green grasses, yarrow, ox-eyed daisy and queen of the meadow. At the base of her great round belly two sacred springs burst forth. One spring surges with water coloured red by rich veins of iron deep within the hills. The other spring flows white with buried calcite formed thousands of years ago from the shells of tiny sea creatures.

Her left breast is the gentle curve of a great hill rising towards the sky. Her vagina lies in the valley's shadow. From the shadow her daughter crowns. Her daughter's emerging head is a hill once called the Bride's Mound, a place where women long ago lived in community, danced and prayed.

Once, long ago, the Birthing-Goddess was bathed in the ocean's salty water and wrapped in mists.

People still gather where her great belly folds into the surrounding flat lands to bathe in the waters flowing from the white spring. They immerse themselves in the waters seeking healing and solace. Some stories tell us that the white waters are the Birthing-Goddess's breast milk, while others say the waters are the creamy white vaginal release that marks her fertility. There are those who believe these are the ancient seawaters, from which we all are born.

The red waters were once bathed in, to heal broken hearts and wounded bodies. They are now covered with a lid decorated with two overlapping circles pierced by a sword. Old stories tell us the red waters symbolize the blood the Goddess sheds as she births her daughter. Others speak of the red waters as menstrual blood. The red spring was once used as a portal to the Birthing-Goddess's womb in ritual to renew life.

Now her hills and valleys have been plowed and planted with fields of hay and are pasture for sheep.

People no longer tell stories of the red water being the blood of the Goddess. It is now the blood of Christ. It is said that the man who buried Christ after he was taken down from the crucifix traveled to the isle of the Birthing-Goddess with a cup of Christ's blood. When he poured the blood into the waters, the spring began to run red, and has done so ever since. Legend has it that the Holy Grail lies deep inside the red running spring.

During the medieval period the Birthing-Goddess's hills and valleys were a favourite place for building great churches and monasteries. The Great Glastonbury Abby was one of the richest and most powerful monasteries in England at one time. All that remains of it now is an imposing tower on the Goddess's left breast called the Tor and within her vagina the ruins of the Lady's Chapel—the sanctuary to the Virgin.

The sea-water that rose as mists over the Goddess, veiling her, were dammed by the Church as its fortune and power grew. The saline waters, rising and falling with the season, were drained away to make way for farm land.

The Bride's Mound, the hill representing the Goddess's emerging daughter, is paved over and hosts an abandoned industrial park and sewage treatment plant.

Scarred by religion and industrialization, when the Moon of Flowering rises bright and round in the month of May, the Birthing-Goddess bursts with the green of spring. All over her hills and deep in her valleys wildflowers dance with bees and butterflies. Her bogs and ditches awaken with marigold's golden yellow and swans nest in her shallow pools.

If you flew over the Birthing-Goddess and looked down over her hills and valleys you would see the shape of an old woman riding a swan flying in a southeasterly direction. In the ancient traditions of the birthing land, it is from the southeast that dreams arrive. The women who have danced since before memory, swirling and circling, celebrating fertility, did not see a man on the face of the Moon, but swans. The graceful beauty is an animal sacred to the Goddess with its neck curving like a snake from the body of a bird. The swans swim in the milky white waters of the Moon, the deep well of the night sky.

The Moon, snakes and swans all teach us the Wisdom of the Great Round: the change that never changes the snake that sheds it skin, the swans that come and go with the change of season. The Moon herself turns towards fullness and then turns to darkness. Like a woman's monthly shedding of blood and her power to bring forth life, these are symbols of nature's eternal rhythms, the coming and going of all of life, again and again.

The phases of the Moon, the sliver of light, the

great white globe and the gentle turning to darkness mirror the rhythms of a woman's fertility, both her monthly cycles and her journey from puberty to crone. The Moon marks the embracing of life and the releasing of life. The changing Moon, a trickle of menstrual blood, swans flight overhead and the empty snake skin are echoes of the change that never changes —the continuous birth, life, death and rebirth cycle of life.

Women and the Moon share rhythms. The Moon's fullness coincides with the release of a woman's egg and the flow of creamy white vaginal fluid. The fluid provides passage for sperm beyond a woman's cervix, the gateway to new life. During the dark Moon, the womb releases blood. In the darkness, the Moon slowly turns again towards fullness. With the letting down of blood, ovaries begin to ripen eggs for another cycle.

Before electricity and maternity wards, most babies were birthed by the light of the full Moon. Moon pushing and pulling the currents of life with waves of contractions old as time, shone a soft light for women to birth new life.

Like the ocean's tides, women are pulled by eternal cycling of the Moon. The Moon brings the light of dreams bursting with creativity and joy. Or it cloaks a woman in darkness. The thin light of the crescent Moon hears her longings and griefs. Who knows how many secrets have been whispered before the Moon? Who knows the many times the Moon has carried women through the stormy seas of life?

I have to wonder if Sarah turned to the Moon when

her husband Abraham took her son up on the mountain with a sharp blade and eyes blazing with vision. But I am ahead of myself. Let's first tell this oldest of stories.

Sarah had been barren for many years when she laughed at the prophet who told her would become pregnant. She had swelled with hope too many times to plunge into the despair of an empty womb. Yet, her belly bloomed and she birthed a boy, strong and healthy. It was so odd to see an old woman with a newborn that her friends, family, and neighbours whispered amongst themselves, "Did she find the child abandoned on the roadside?"

To put an end to the gossip, Sarah and Abraham invited all they knew to a feast. During the feast, Sarah breastfed all the infants who arrived with their mothers. After that, everyone knew Sarah was the boy's birth mother. She named her son Isaac.

After many years of mothering her only precious child, a terrible vision was revealed to her husband, Abraham. In the vision Abraham's God, who had blessed him with great wealth and promises of future prosperity, demanded a blood sacrifice of Isaac—their precious son.

Imagine Sarah's distress when Abraham, the man to whom she had been bound for most of her life, a fanatic with inspired purpose, cast her aside to fulfill his God's cruel desire.

Now, Sarah could not stop herself from pummelling Abraham's back with her fists, an ungodly cry pouring from her heart as he sharpened his knife. Sarah begged and pleaded, wept and wailed, threatened and cursed, implored her husband to forsake his God and spare her son. Abraham, deaf to her pain, offered no compassion to sooth the torrent of despair that consumed Sarah's heart. Abraham was compelled to follow his God who promised greatness. Isaac's life was the price to be paid for Abraham's desires.

After Abraham turned away with his knife and her son, Sarah stumbled into the streets desperate to find her husband and save her son. In her fear and grief, she beseeched neighbours and street vendors, housewives and strangers, pleading, "Have you seen Abraham? Which way did he turn?"

When news that Abraham had sacrificed a ram and her son still lived reached her, Sarah clenched her heart, collapsed and with a soft moan died in the street.

The traditional way this story is told is that Isaac laid down on the rock baring his throat and as Abraham ran his finger along the edge the blade testing its sharpness an angel appeared. The angel directed Abraham's gaze to a ram caught in the thorns of a thicket. Seeing the ram, Abraham understood it was a sign from God to spare his son. He caught the ram and sacrificed it instead. The shrub that caught the ram was Vitex agnus-castus.

The curator of Neot Kedumim Botanical Garden in Israel, Dr. Sarah Oren, writes that Vitex was the plant that the ram was tangled in. Vitex's botanical name still carries the essence of this cruel story. Translated from Latin the word agnus means "lamb", castus means "purity".

Let's take a look at the story of Sarah, Abraham and Isaac with another light—the light of the Moon.

In a temple on the Isle of Crete, a place sacred to the Goddess Cere The Earth Mother, women decorated temples with Vitex's blossoms. The women who decorated Cere's temple were mothers. They were not wistful virgins nor wizened crones. They were women in the fullness of their lives. Their stomachs were no longer flat, their breasts were soft from nursing and snaking scars shimmered across their bellies where life had swelled. The women hung garlands of Vitex's violet flowers, in gratitude for the medicine the thorny shrub offered their bodies as they flowed with the Moon's waxing, fullness, waning and darkness.

Vitex, a plant ruled by the Moon, helps a woman's cycle rise and fall with the Moon. It eases the pain of bleeding. It quickens the release of an egg. It keeps a baby quiet, if restless to leave the womb. Vitex softens a girl's transition to womanhood, and supports a woman's release into the life of a crone. Vitex supports the change that is always on its way.

The ram that caught Abraham's eye was trapped by the thorns of a Vitex bush, a plant ruled by the Moon and known to support a woman in her love for her children. This tells us the old tale can be told another way.

Before being gifted to Abraham, Sarah's name was Sarai and her people lived high in the mountains of what is now Iraq. During Sarai's life this land was infused with Sumerian culture. Sumerians like Sarai's family worshipped the Moon God Nanna. The Moon was a God of great wisdom. As the Moon, Nanna watched over women in their birthing. Nanna the Moon God was a guardian of mothers.

Anguished by her husband's God's demand for the blood of her son, did Saria turn to Moon, the God of her childhood? Did the Moon hear the inconsolable grief in Sarai's prayers? Did Nanna offer a ram for Abraham's blood-thirsty God? Did the Moon tangle up the ram in Vitex's thorns—a bush ruled by the Moon carrying medicine that supports a mother's love for her child?

God knows women need support with their hormone cycles, particularly since he laid down a curse on every woman since Eve, "To the woman He said: "I will greatly multiply your sorrow and your conception; In pain you shall bring forth children; Your desire shall be for your husband, And he shall rule over you." (Genesis 3:16) Later God announced:

> When a woman has a discharge, and the discharge in her body is blood, she shall be in her menstrual impurity for seven days, and whoever touches her shall be unclean until the evening. And everything on which she lies during her menstrual impurity shall be unclean. Everything also on which she sits shall be unclean. And whoever touches her bed shall wash his clothes and bathe himself in water and be unclean until the evening. And whoever touches anything on which she sits shall wash his clothes and bathe himself in water and be unclean until the evening. Whether it is the bed or anything on which she sits,

> when he touches it, he shall be unclean until the evening. (Leviticus 15:19-30)

AND THE CURSING OF A WOMEN'S FERTILITY CYCLE continued throughout the ages. Pliny the Elder, a Roman scholar whose writings were the scientific authority throughout the Middle Ages was one of the few to write about menstruating women.

> If the menstrual discharge coincides with an eclipse of the moon or sun, the evils resulting from it are irremediable; and no less so, when it happens while the moon is in conjunction with the sun; the congress with a woman at such a period being noxious and attended with fatal effects to the man.
>
> As well as bees, it is a well-known fact, will forsake their hives if touched by a menstruous woman; that linen boiling in the cauldron will turn black, that the edge of a razor will become blunted, and that copper vessels will contract a fetid smell and become covered with Verdi grease, on coming in contact with her. A mare big with foal, if touched by a woman in this state, will be sure to miscarry; nay, even more than this, at the very sight of a woman. (Pliny the Elder. Natural History).

Pliny the Elder also attributed strange medicinal attributes to menstrual blood which included curing rabies and intermittent fevers as well as tumours, boils, and ulcers.

Beliefs about destructive forces attributed to a woman's fertility cycle, teachings of its inherent sinfulness has caused shamefulness to seep into everyday understanding of a woman's monthly bleed.

When I was growing up my mother alternated between calling the menstrual cycle a curse or a friend. I think it depended on whether or not she had had sex that month. After her fifth child, she did not want or need more children.

I remember boys in high school snickering at a girl "on the rag".

Once a boyfriend of mine complained about the bloody disgusting smell of the woman sitting next to him on the bus. He was sure she had her period.

I recall sitting in the girls' change room in middle school and the gym teacher offering advice on how to secretly bleed. It involved wearing dark coloured clothing and intensive hygiene protocols. I remember carefully rolling up tampons in wades of toilet paper, hiding the evidence that I was bleeding and hoping no one could smell me.

Advertising on pads and tampons have cashed in on a woman's monthly shame.

Throughout the early 1900's Lysol made its money telling women to douche with Lysol or else their husbands might leave them because of the smell of their vaginas. In 1911, 5 deaths and 193 poisonings were recorded by women douching with Lysol. Lysol did not stop promoting its noxious household cleanser for douching until the Pill became available in the mid '60's.

In the 1920's pads were promoted as a solution to a woman's 'intimate problem'. From the 40's to the 70's, the top selling brand of pads and tampons was called "Modest". Today pads, tampons and cups are still described as "discrete" and "undetectable" by advertisers. An ad for scented panty liners in 2014 suggested their product was a good choice if a woman cannot stay in the shower all day.

In the 1990's advertising assured women using a tampon would not disturb their virginity. In 2015, a new product for feminine hygiene came on the market called Softcup that promised no leakage for 12 hours. Their advertising inferred that a woman could have sex using their product and her partner would never know she was bleeding.

Herbalists spend lots of time talking about how exogenous estrogen, including plastics and pesticides, disturb a woman's cycle. Herbalists regularly discuss the effects of stress on a woman's cycle and recommend herbs called adaptogens to moderate cortisol levels in order to rebalance the menstrual cycle. But we rarely speak of the generations of shame projected on a woman's fertility cycle and the effects shame has on the woman's physical and mental health.

Think about it. If you are told repeatedly by men and women, advertising promotions, and your religious and educational institutions that the blood passing from your uterus every month is bad, stinks, shameful, disgusting, sinful, cursed, something to hide etc., it seems unlikely you are going to feel good while bleeding.

As an herbalist, the most common health challenges I am presented with are some sort of female hormonal imbalance. Irregular hormones cause significant physical, emotional, mental and spiritual pain for women of all ages. Their lives are disrupted. Their dreams and talents are undermined.

For some, hormonal imbalance leads to committing violent crimes, forced hospitalization in psychiatric institutions, and untimely death. (https://pubmed.ncbi.nlm.nih.gov/2062202/)

Hormonal imbalances cause cramps, scarring acne, endometriosis, polycystic ovary syndrome (PCOs), infertility, fibroids, migraines, thyroid disorders, premenstrual dystrophic disorder (PDMM), as well as cervical, breast and uterine cancer. That is just to name a few.

Let's return to our Birthing-Goddess amongst the hills in Glastonbury, England and the Moon's ever-changing face gazing down on her. The Moon and the Birthing-Goddess have been partnered in their dance with light and darkness, barrenness and fertility for a long time.

The dance between the Moon and its pull on the Earth's water is older than Pliny the Elder's superstitions, older than the stories of the curse Eve carried, older than Abraham's knife. The Goddess, or should I say, the Earth Mother, responds to the ever-changing light of the Moon. Walk in the forest during the dark Moon and feel Nature's stillness as she pauses in anticipation of Moon's return. During dark Moon Nature's dance is suspended as the next steps are dreamt.

Walk in the forest under the full moon and feel the magic as trees sway with blue Moon shadows and owls call from somewhere near and far. The forest welcomes the light and the dark of the Moon.

A woman's body is a sequence of Earth's steps in its dance to Moon's rhythms of ever-changing light. The dance is a woman's shifting mood as her womb fills, reaches fullness, overflows and becomes empty. The Moon mirrors the stages of a woman's womb: the virginal, fertile and barren. Becoming aware, dancing with Moon and Earth brings peacefulness to the never-ending cycle of birth, life, death and rebirth, a cycle reflected in a woman's menarche, monthly bleed, pregnancy and menopause.

Vitex helps women relearn the steps to this ancient fertility dance. Understanding that women's bodies do not need to be sanitized, perfumed, disguised or controlled brings calm to the heart and feelings of rooted belonging. Vitex supports a woman's body in finding the Moon's rhythm. Vitex opens a woman to the wisdom of the flow inherent in ending and beginnings.

Even though we live in a world with 24-hour lighting and indoor heating, push button shopping and hot water on demand, there is no getting away from the rhythms of our bodies. Satiation follows hunger. Sleep follows fatigue. Restfulness follows sleep. Bowels need to be emptied after a meal. Lungs need to fill after exhalation. Cold seeks heat and heat seeks cold. To have a body is to be fated to fulfill its many corporeal needs or else live with the consequences, at best feeling tired and grumpy, at worse seriously ill.

A woman's body carries a deeper yearning than eating, shitting and sleeping. Women carry a yearning that comes and goes with the fullness of the Moon, the flow of blood and the passing of years. It is a yearning that irrevocably marks a woman's life. The yearning for a child tugs at a woman's womb, pulls on her mind and wrenches her heart.

So many women have said to me, "I never thought I wanted children, till now." Or, "Who knew I would be so happy to be pregnant." Or, "I never knew I could love like this."

It is as if a women's need for a child is driven by forces beyond understanding. A woman and her fertility often seems fated. Whether a woman births a child or many children, births a still child or births no children, miscarries, adopts or chooses abortions, a mark is left behind on her womb and her heart. The mark is like a story whose true meaning can never be revealed with words or images. The mark carries a silent uncertainty and tenderness for life.

The life blood a woman bleeds each cycle of the Moon, the children she births or does not birth, her power to carry life, bring her wisdom. It is not surprising the Fates, the most ancient of Goddesses wise in the coming into being and passing away of life, were known to weave the threads that bind soul to flesh by the light of the Moon.

Conception, even with today's technological methods of conceiving a child, is mysterious. Sometimes it works. Sometimes it doesn't. Often there is no explanation why some women are as fertile as the sea, while others no matter how their heart pleads for a child, remain barren. It does not matter if conception is an unexpected surprise, a well-planned coupling or it never arrives, conception of a child feels like a decision made by the Fates.

Pregnancy takes control of a woman's body, emotions and mind. Every part of a woman's life is touched by pregnancy: her mood, bowel movements, cravings, sleep, libido, self-esteem, dreams. Some women love being pregnant. Others hate it. Every woman is surprised by the experience, whether pleasurable or riddled with suffering. No two pregnancies are the same. During pregnancy, a woman's body, mind and soul are in the hands of the Fates as they weave within her womb, flesh and soul into the shape of a child.

Birth is the moment when the Fates demand a woman completely let go. In ancient times when women birthed by the light of the full Moon, the Fates were offered bread. Midwives sang as they held the woman in her labour, "May this child and mother live through this night to see the dawn".

Birth is a twilight time when women hover between life and death. To the ancients, it was the most fated of moments in a life. Prayers to the Moon were offered as it tugged on the womb's tides, the embryonic sea, until they overflowed the boundaries of the womb and washed ashore a child, naked and hungry.

When there is no pregnancy and the Moon vanishes from the night sky, the hand of the great goddess Hecate, the Goddess of the dark Moon and crossroads, grips a woman's heart and wrenches out the poison of anger, resentment, betrayal and bitterness until her womb bleeds thick bloody clots of wrath. Or, Hecate with her sharpened blade nicks a woman's heart and in seeps the sorrows of the world, dying hopes and dreams, while warm sticky blood is felt on the inner thigh and the cleansing begins. Sometimes the woman is washed with relief for she did not want the child made from the seed of a man who did not love her as she should be loved.

I have listened to many stories birthed in wombs—fearful tales of pushing to no end, labours that are brutal, demeaning, and frightening. I have heard the secrets of miscarriages and fetus' bloody on white bed sheets. I have listened to abortion's shame and regret. I have watched women seeking a child cling to a thin thread of hope laced with ultra-sounds and gloved hands, needles in bellies, only to end in more gushing blood. I have heard sobbing stories, angry stories, confused stories. Women who are smart, kind, aware tell stories of losing control while rage and sorrow toss them about like a ship lost at sea. I have heard the bitterness of betrayals, waiting too long and the despair of regret. I have sat with women while their newborns struggle for breath in a plastic box and their breasts leak with milk-like tears. I have listened to women who thought they had a choice, only to discover that the choice to conceive or not to conceive, to birth or not to birth is fated.

I have not met a woman whose life has not been shaped, no matter her intentions, beliefs or goodness, by the flux of her hormones driven by the Moon's waxing and waning and her ability to carry the weaving of the Fates.

But we never speak of Fate these days. The Earth Mother is a resource and storage facility, not a living body birthing life each spring and gathering back life each fall. As for the Moon—man has landed on it. It is nothing but a rock. Perhaps it might become a useful mining exposition.

Technological and biomedical medicine has tossed aside the ancient Goddesses weaving by the well of the Moon. Women are no longer fated to bleed with birth control that stops the flow. Bio-identical hormones slow the thinning of skin, hair and vaginal walls. It seems like we have transcended the shame of Biblical times, and superstitions of the Middle Ages. We haven't.

I still see girls blush when asked if they have begun their monthly bleeding. They watch their mothers pretend they are not bleeding as they rush off to work, pick up sons at hockey and grab a few groceries. Few know what to say when babies are stillborn . Women do not speak of abortions. Miscarriages are silent. And, after a dreadfully traumatic labour, women often feel it is wrong to weep for days with their bundle of joy.

Then one night unable to sleep, after pretending, silencing and trying to be all that she thinks she should be, a woman gazes at the Moonlight streaming through the window and says, “I feel dead inside”. These four words awaken an ancient ancestral voice from deep within her womb.

Arriving in my office, she’ll say, “I don’t know what made me call an herbalist. I don’t even know what you do.” And she tells me her womb’s story and I tell her about Vitex, a plant ruled by the Moon.

Vitex, a tiny berry about the size of the pituitary gland, can change a woman’s life.

Where there was no bleeding with the turn of the Moon, Vitex awakens a woman’s fertility cycle. When a woman bleeds to exhaustion, Vitex slows the bleeding and returns vitality. Vitex guides women gracefully through menopause and leads a girl into womanhood. Vitex calms the spasms of miscarriage, brings light into the heart of postpartum depression and lets down breast milk. Vitex eases migraines and stills restless nights. Vitex is a plant that lifts the curse: the rage, the weeping, the gushing blood and pain. Vitex restores balance to a woman’s fertility cycle, releasing her into the timeless cycle of life without shame, regret and hopelessness.

I often wonder what a woman’s life would be like if she was not taught to hide the blood she sheds each month. Would raging be calmed and weeping be soothed? Would pain be relieved and gushing be slowed? Would the yearning for a child be heard? Would the loss of miscarriage be tended to? What would happen if a young girl was told from a very young age that she carried a sacred power—the gift to weave a life?

The Celts believed that menstrual blood carried

wisdom. When the wisdom blood was no longer shed, it pulsed through a woman's veins and she became wise. The Moon carries the wisdom of the eternal change that never changes. This is the wisdom of monthly bleeding—beginnings birthed by endings, and endings seeded in beginnings.

The Celts journeyed to the land where the Birth-Goddess lay and bathed in her red spring to heal curses and wounds. In the spring the Celts collected her red waters and sprinkled it over their fields while asking for her blessings on the soil they tilled.

The Celts lived in a time when a woman's ability to birth a child was sacred. They traced her blood each month to the cycling of the Moon and the rise and fall of the tides. They understood that a woman's body carries the same sacred creative life force that stretches the ewe's belly in the early spring, brings blossoms to the apple tree, ripens the wheat gold, and sculpts the pumpkin's voluptuous curves. They knew it was the Moon that set the course for the seeding, ripening and passing of life.

The Moon teaches it is only from the darkness that one is reborn. The Moon offers the light and the darkness for the dance women have danced since beyond memory.

MERCURY, VOLFA, AND VALERIAN

> There was in the settlement the woman whose name was Thorbjorg. She was a prophetess (spa-queen) and was called Litilvolva. She had had nine sisters, and they were all spa-queens, and she was the only one now living. It was a custom of Thorbjorg, in the wintertime, to make a circuit, and people invited her into their houses, especially those who had any curiosity about the season, or desired to know their fate....(Dashu. 2017.)

The sun was setting when the Volfa appeared. She stood in the doorway crooked and bent, draped in a dark blue cloak studded with gemstones glistening like stars. Her ice blue eyes gazed into our gentle home. A chill scurried across the floor and settled into the gloom lurking in the corners.

Her hand gloved in a cat's soft white fur pushed the hood of her cloak back. Her skin, finely lined, was as thin as the wisps of mist that rise from river in moonlight. The broad curve of her cheekbones was easily traced by the eye. On her head she wore the fur of a black lamb trimmed with the skin of a white cat. In the crook of her arm, she held her staff of sturdy iron. A metal distaff was welded to the top. Rings hung from the distaff and sprinkled her every movement with tinkling music like firefly's spark in night darkness.

I am left to wonder about these Mercurial women, the Spa Queens also called the Volfu, who wandered through the Northern European winter practicing prophesy. Spa-queens have many names and the designation of each is lost in time but here are a few: Spakona which is translated into Spa-queen is derived from Spakona – spa meaning prophesy and Kona meaning woman. Or Volfa – also Volva- meaning wise woman or prophetess. Volfu is the plural of Volfa.

There is little known about them. Some nasty poetry recites stories about groups of men publicly stoning, burning or piercing them with spears and the Volfus' tenacious power to be reborn and go on to offer healing ceremonies for their communities.

Some poetry even accuses the Volfu of being the joy of evil women.

From their unearthed graves the tools of the Volfas' trade have been extracted. Their bones have been dug up as far west as Ireland and as far east as Russia, in places colonized by the Norse. Most of their graves have been disturbed in Norway, Sweden and Denmark.

With their bones lay a wand, or a staff depending on the writer reporting the disinterment. I prefer to think of a Volfa carrying a staff as opposed to a wand. Staffs seem steadier, a close friend to lean on as the Volfa walked from village to village wrapped in furs as protection against the bone chilling wind that howls across the North Sea.

Mercury also carries a staff. Mercury is neither he nor she although most frequently referred to in the masculine. Mercury uses her staff to rouse the sleeping or to send those awake into deep sleep. Mercury's staff offers a gentle death or helps return the dead to the land of the living.

Fascinating as the Volfu's unearthed staffs are, their silent graves do not reveal their healing songs and the plants they used.

Amongst the bones of one Volfa was a pouch containing Henbane seeds. This was at the time a commonly used psychoactive European plant. The Norse planted sacred gardens with Henbane. The plant was used for divination, for changing the weather, and for finding treasure. There is no doubt a Volfa was trained in making mead with the magical plant and using it in ceremony.

But to serve in a communal ceremony with the gift of prophesy, the Volfa would need to be alert. Powerfully psychoactive plants may have been better suited for personal ceremonies or ceremonies for the initiated. As communities contain all sorts of different types of people, the Volfa may have wanted to keep one foot planted on this side of the veil in case disturbing beliefs threatened her harm while she publicly called upon the dead.

The ceremony the Volfa offered the communities

strung out along the old paths through the hills and valleys of Northern Europe was call seidr. During the seidr, the Volva called upon the dead to help weave a future free of strife, hunger and heartbreak for the living. I do not pretend to know how the ancient ceremony of seidr proceeded. Yet my curiosity calls me to imagine the darkness of the room, the flicker of candle light, the pungent smoke of herbs and the melody of the songs as the Volfa crossed the veil between the living and the dead on a cold winter's night. I let my imagination play as I call forth the seidr and ask Mercury to guide me in catching the Volfa's seidr on the wind while mingling fact with fiction.

My simple prayer was, "May Mercury and her gift with words thread the Volva's story and her ways through the thin eye of the needle poised between the darkness of the past and the darkness of the future."

Silence creeps. Once, not long ago, green leaves whispered rain's song in warm breezes and bees returned home with heavy sacs of brightly coloured pollen clinging to their back legs, while bird music pierced warm evening's crimson skies as Moon rose and Sun set. Now stillness falls across the land as skeletal branches scrap the grey sky and the veil between the worlds thins.

We had spent days preparing for her and the guests she calls to us on this night. We scrubbed the floors, slaughtered the animals and mixed their bones with twigs and branches in preparation for the great bonfire. My mother made a special stew for the Volfa from the hearts of each animal slaughtered. It bubbled all day over the fire before it was extinguished. We set the table with a feast of roast lamb, squash stuffed with sweet nuts, sturdy loafs of dense bread and baked apples.

As we kneaded the dense bread to be served at the feast, my mother had urged me clarify my private thoughts and wishes. My first blood had appeared when the raspberry ripened this past summer. I am now old enough to ask the Volva a question from my heart and also to choose a husband.

When all was prepared, the fire was extinguished. In the darkness with cold creeping into our home, we sat waiting for the guests.

My mother gasped at the sight of the Volva in our doorway: an old woman cloaked in the colour of midnight, wisps of frost-covered hair escaping beneath her hat of fur and a steely gaze that peered into each of our faces as if seeking to know more than any stranger should. My mother did not breathe until the old woman held out her hand in friendly greeting as one of her girls removed her cloak. Beneath it she wore a red dress woven from nettle fibres and around her waist was a belt with a pouch made from the polypore that grows on the birch tree. In the pouch, she carried her magic plants.

While the Volva probably carried with her Henbane and other psychoactive gifts from nature, such as Psilocybin, I suspect roots of Valerian (Valerianna officinalis) were also tucked away for safe keeping in the pouch she carried on her hip. Valerian is a herb whose name has sprung from the same root as the word valour. The Volfa had to have a brave heart to do the work of seidr.

Let's spiral forward to modern day and explore the mysteries of Valerian, a plant ruled by Mercury the Psychopomp, a guide for the souls of the dead. Mercury, the planet, also governs healers and shamans.

A few years ago, at an herb gathering on Vancouver Island I was sitting around with a group of practicing herbalists sharing stories about hypnotics, herbs for sleep. Everyone agreed Valerian is not always reliable. The consensus was it's too tricky and spontaneous. After offering Valerian for sleep, we had all had the call the next day from a weary client complaining that the plant had kept them awake with weird thoughts and restlessness. Unreliable Valerian, ruled by the unpredictable trickster Mercury, keeps even the most seasoned herbalist guessing.

At another herb gathering in Arizona, I met an herbalist who gave advice on how to tame this wily plant. There are two parts to this understanding.

The first part is that Valerian carries a spark of fire. The energy of fire is warming and rises. The fire in Valerian rises to the head. In other words, it increases circulation of blood in thc brain. This can also be attributed to its effect on the adenosine receptor sites found in the brain. But more on that later.

The second part is that Valerian is also ruled by Mercury, the chatty planet. An increase in the fire element mingled with Mercury's chatty vibration creates medicine that is contra-indicted for overthinkers. It keeps them awake thinking.

Valerian is better suited to the individual who is at a loss for words. This is the person who lies in bed at night awake without a thought in her head. Valerian helps these people both sleep and find their lost words. Mercury rules speech.

The other medicine Valerian offers calms spasms. It is an anti-spasmodic.

Once I gave Valerian to a woman who was diagnosed with interstitial cystitis with painful bladder spasms that kept her awake at night. I recommended she take 10 drops of Valerian just before bed. It worked like a charm. With a small dose of Valerian, the spasms disappeared. Over a couple of months, Valerian cured the spasms all together.

Interestingly, this woman was also having difficulty experiencing orgasm. Valerian also cured this problem. It is a traditional aphrodisiac.

So, when my Mom, who struggles with insomnia and lies in bed all night not thinking, began to experience bladder spasms I gave her Valerian 10 drops before bed to take.

With Valerian's care the spasms disappeared, and she, in her own words "slept like a teenager". My Mom was so happy with Valerian's effects she began to encourage her friends to take Valerian. Try to explain to your Mother that herbal medicine is not the same as over the counter medicine.

All was well for about two months. Then, in the late fall my Mom's life-long friend, who had passed away six months earlier visited her.

"She was standing at the foot of my bed wearing the

coat we bought in Woolworths when we were 16." There was an edge to my Mom's voice.

"Maybe she wants to tell you something," I suggested scrolling through my emails, half listening to her strange story. My Mom is full of stories.

"I am not interested in talking to dead people," and the subject was closed.

A couple of nights later, my Mom woke up and went into the kitchen to get a glass of water to find children in her living room. This perked up my ears. I know, from working in a hospice, people often see children in the week or so before they pass.

"What were they doing?" I asked.

"Just playing," she said. She was less upset about the children than she was about her friend's visitation.

A couple of nights later, something happened that completely freaked my Mom out. My Mom lives in a seniors' building. On this particular night, just as the last leaves fell from the trees, she woke up to find all the people from her building who had died in the past 10 years streaming into her bedroom.

"They were all complaining about how they had been treated in their final years," her voice carried the high pitch of panic.

I was stumped. I have always known my Mom has some uncanny abilities. But she had never had such intense experiences of mediumship. Then she told me, "It's your fault this is happening."

"My fault!"

"It's that Valerian bringing all these dead people to

me!" She had poured it down the toilet just before calling me.

Curious, I called up one of my experienced plant friends and asked her if she had ever heard of Valerian being used for mediumship. My friend confirmed my Mom's experience.

There are scientific papers suggesting experiences of ghosts take place in the brain and not in creepy old houses, graveyards and morgues. The research suggests some brains are more prone to experiencing ghosts. These brains have irregularly functioning temporal lobes, particularly the right lobe. (Persinger. 2001).

While the left temporal lobe is involved in language, learning and recalling verbal information, the right lobe gives the ability to understand and learn non-verbal information such as music and visual-spatial material and stuff you remember seeing, like a plant or face. The right temporal lobe of your brain is also sensitive to shifts in the electrical magnetic field (EMF).

The EMF is the weaving of the Earth's naturally occurring electricity and its magnetic field. NASA explains the magnetic field this way.

> The magnetic field of Earth is caused by currents of electricity that flow in the molten core. These currents are hundreds of miles wide and flow at thousands of miles per hour as the Earth rotates. The powerful magnetic field passes out through the core of Earth, passes through the crust and enters space. (Odenwold. 2003).

THE EARTH'S MAGNETIC FIELD IS PROFOUNDLY influenced by the Sun. The Sun's magnetic field pushes against the Earth's field. When the Earth turns to face the Sun during daytime, the Earth's magnetic field is pushed out the side of the Earth facing away from the sun. During the night, all of life living on the surface of the Earth is infused with higher levels of the Earth's magnetism than during the day.

The rotation of the Earth also influences the strength of the Earth's magnetic field. It only goes to reason then, that as the nights become longer in the Northern Hemisphere the influence of the EMFs strengthens.

People who experience ghosts tend to have right temporal lobes sensitive to shifts in the EMF. This may be caused by an accident, seizures, mental illness (schizophrenics have sensitive right temporal lobes) and infection and plants like Valerian. When the days lengthen, those with sensitive right temporal lobes become more open to otherworldly experiences. It is not surprising our ancestors chose late October, early November to welcome the dead into their homes for a feast and ask them for guidance.

Valerian is a nighttime herb. In all my years as an herbalist I can count on the fingers of one hand the number of times I have put it in a formula for use during the day. Whether to calm spasms or support sleep, it almost always is added to formulas taken in the evening as the sun goes down.

At low doses, Valerian eases spasms and supports sleep. At higher doses it causes excitation and people, like my mother, experience visits from the dead. The plant has these effects by shifting the neurochemistry in the temporal lobes, particularly the right.

We know Valerian influences, by mimicking, two different neurotransmitters. The first is GABA (Gamma aminobutyric acid), a calm, easy-going neurotransmitter that opens one to the flow of life. Herbs that increase the GABA in the brain, like Valerian, Passionflower and Kava, are used when people struggle with higher than usual levels of anxiety.

These herbs also support sleep. Herbalists have a long history of using these herbs to decrease the number and intensity of epileptic seizures associated with the right temporal lobe.

The second known neurotransmitter Valerian mimics is adenosine, a neurotransmitter that slows the body and the mind down. This is the neurotransmitter that increases blood flow to the brain. The neurotransmitter adenosine is calming and is necessary for us to journey into sleep.

And here we meet the vibration of Mercury. If Valerian only inhibited the re-uptake of calming GABA to create a go-with-the-flow attitude in life, or only acted upon adenosine quieting down states of arousal, herbalists would not consider Valerian a tricky herb. It would be a plant that guaranteed a good night's sleep, and it would probably have been given over to the Moon and not Mercury for rulership.

Precisely how Valerian affects the brain, we may

never know. No matter how much pharmaceutical companies try, plant medicine can't be reduced to single phytoconstituents interacting with cells' receptors. Plants are not simpletons; they are intelligent.

A plant ruled by Mercury is intelligent and will defy reductionistic beliefs about validating only measurable experiences.

Mercury the messenger of the Gods knows that Gods are fickle, and their messages change with their moods. Mercury is not attached to the message she brings. Mercury flows in whatever direction the wind blows. Mercury is non-binary. Mercury is neither male nor female but open to all other possible genders. Mercury doesn't just communicate with the living, but also the dead and everything in between. Mercury, while loving logic, relies on intuition, picking up subtle information riding on the wind, or perhaps shifts in the Earth's magnetic frequency. It is easy to see why Mercury also rules the brain. The brain is the trickiest organ in the body. It is easy to see why herbalists/astrologers gave Valerian the rulership of Mercury, a plant that shifts the brain's experience of reality.

In the 1990's neuroscientists invented what they called God's Helmet and likened it to the helmet the Roman's version of Mercury wore. Putting on God's Helmet allowed scientists to send different types of electrical signals into temporal lobes. Some of these signals mimicked frequencies produced by the Earth's magnetic field. Most of the subjects, when their temporal lobes were stimulated with EMF like signals, experienced a presence or, in other words, a ghost.

Therefore, it has been decided that ghosts are caused in electrical disturbances to the temporal lobe. These researchers suggested that those who experience ghosts and other worldly energies suffer with some sort of temporal brain disorder that causes excessive sensitivity to EMFs.

I would suggest that these neuroscientists while using their mercurial intelligence to design a novel helmet that shifted a human's perception, lacked Mercury's intellectual dexterity when summing up the results of their studies. Who is to say that the electrical current created by the helmet did not enhance the subject's perceptive ability to experience a presence that was already there but could not be experienced with ordinary sensing abilities?

I am sure the ancestors gathered in the dark room waiting for the Volva to perform the seidr knew the answer to that question. For without plants like Valerian, ruled by Mercury the Psychopomp to enhance one's sensitivity to EMFs and perception of the otherworld, the ceremony that welcomes the dead and asks for their guidance may not have been possible.

Now back to our story.

The day of the ceremony the Volfa and her women rest. Only the woman who speaks with plants moves about our home preparing the herbs used for the night's ritual. She brews a pot of Valerian.

As it quietly simmers over the fire, its strong scent fills the house. Cats, in their daytime slumber catch a whiff of the sacred plant's medicine and awaken. They rub against the legs of the plant woman, bawling their otherworld songs, calling to the ecstasy the plant offers them. I am crouched in a corner near the woman quietly watching when she turns to me and tells me the cats are infusing their night seeing medicine into the bubbling brew.

Beside the decocting Valerian, the plant woman prepares herbs to be burned. Their smoke will aid the Volva in her journey. As the Sun sets, she fills small iron pots with the herbs to be burnt. She strains the Valerian root from the decoction she tended to all day and pours it into a large silver bowl the Volfa brought with her. She takes the roots outside and buries them at the foot of an ash tree.

When the Sun sets below the horizon, the fire in the hearth is put out. Darkness fills all spaces. The air is thick with the smoke of Mugwort, Yarrow and Valerian. Silence with not even a restless shuffling of feet fills the room. The Volva whispers into the silver bowl containing Valerian's medicine, calling on Valerian's medicine using the plant's old names, Cat Weed and Moon Root.

There stands an ash I know
called Yggdrasil
a mighty tree moist with shining drops
from it come dew that fall adown
it stands green over Urd's well.
Thence come the all-knowing maidens
three in the hall under the tree
Urd is one called, another Verdandi-
they scored the wood – and Skuld the third
they lay down laws, they allot life

from humankind's children, speaking Fates.
(Dashu. 2017).

SHE DRINKS IT. THE WOMEN BEGIN TO SING.

Theirs is a sweet, haunting song with no words to carry meaning. The intoned sounds ride a melody older than time. The women's song sends threads, like currents spiralling in a river, to pull the souls of the ancestors closer to the shores of this world. The melody casts into the vast darkness of the night a net to catch the souls of the dead. Caught in the weave of the song those who dwell below and those who dwell above enter into our world.

When the ancestors are gathered, the prepared feast is offered to them. The women continue to sing as the invisible guests enjoy the taste of the harvest. When it is time, the Volva quietly taps her staff on the floor, and we know we may now ask the questions that stir deep in our hearts. These are questions that carry the hopes and fears of the year to come.

Will disease come this year? If so, what plants should we use?

Will I have a child this year? If so, whom should I name it for?

Should we journey from home this year? If so in what direction will bring the greatest reward?

Who will die? Who will be lost? Who will be found?

And when I ask, who will I marry this year? The Volva responds, "You will not. Your fate is not to marry. Your fate is to journey with me." In the darkness, I feel my mother's hand reach for mine. Her hold is tight.

When the questions have all been asked the women begin to sing again. This song is no longer soft. It carries anguish. It is a wailing cry, loud and coarse. The song's pain I feel in my heart. The Volva's song calls to the lost souls, those who died in violence, confusion or aloneness. These restless souls follow the living. Some draw on a loved one's life force like a dog chewing on a bone, sucking the marrow. My sister begins to weep and moan with a horrible mournful sound like the sea at midnight as a storm comes ashore. The sea swallowed her husband last spring.

My Aunt, her son's skull crushed under the hooves of a horse during a raid this past summer, shakes and trembles, her arms flaying about like one crawling through wet mud.

The neighbour, a kindly woman, begins to growl, gnashing her teeth, the terrible sounds of hunger. Her boy went into the woods just a month ago and has yet to return.

The air is cold. Chills creep across my skin. The singing becomes shrill. The song is frightening. The wind screeches and howls rattling the shutters over the windows. The Volva thumps her staff onto the floor like thunder. Then there is silence. Peace fills the darkness. The weeping, gnashing and trembling stop. We sit together for a long time in the silent darkness.

One more time the Volva thumps her staff on the floor and now we shout and bang the floor with our hands. Some are banging iron pots and bowls with wooden spoons. We send the ancestors back across the veil to the other side.

Outside, the wood and animal bones are set ablaze. We drink mead made from springtime's roses and Mugwort's moon coloured leaves. We dance, the wild dance of release. As morning light begins to dim the stars, we light torches with the fire from last year's bones to carry home. From the torch we light once more the fire in the hearth. We sleep with no fear, no sorrow, no worry.

In the late afternoon, my mother wakes me. We prepare a pack of the warmest wool cloth. She shows me where in my cloak she has sown charms to keep me safe. When the Volva leaves as night falls, I follow her.

MERCURY, DEATH, AND MANDRAKE

Human beings comfortably dwell on the surface of the Earth. Far beneath our feet unfathomable lava beds flow and a solid core of iron hums. We delight in Sunlight skimming across lakes, ponds, rivers while feeling uncertain about the shadowy movements of swaying weeds just below the water's surface. We shudder gazing upon the ocean's dark brooding swirling waves that cover unknowable depths. We call the sky, its twinkling stars and drifting clouds, a ceiling. Images from telescopes show us the sky is not a surface but just the beginning of the incomprehensible. When looking at each other, we see skin, hair and nails—all surfaces of the body. For some of us, the surface of appearance is enough.

Appearances are not enough for curious humans. Some humans follow caves' hollow echoes deep into the Earth where lungs fill with hot, moist air and impenetrable darkness confuses time and space. Some dive through ocean's surface and wonder at the dazzling colours of fish swirling in a singular motion while water's weight threatens to crush human ribs and flood lungs. Humans launch space telescopes anticipating insights beyond the dark surface of the night sky. Others have the courage to peer into another's eyes and catch a glimpse of the light entwined with flesh called the soul. There are restless brave humans who seek gaps in the surface of everyday ordinariness hoping to uncover the mysteries of life, death, healing and illness. All these curious and clever humans are guided by Mercury. Mercury penetrates surfaces like water trickles through cracks in a cement foundation.

To cross surfaces requires cunning and skill, a bit of luck, and more than a few tricks up one's sleeve. Mercury has all this and more. She is a shape-shifter, a trickster and the guardian of thieves. Mercury is also the guardian of healers. Like a good thief, a healer slips into places unnoticed and leaves behind a sense that something has changed, but what that something is remains uncertain. A skilled healer shifts and shapes the space she works in and has many secret devices in her medicine bag. Guided by Mercury, a healer coaxes another to cross the wide divide between illness and health without noticing the journey laid out before them.

Mercury is also the messenger. And like any messenger, Mercury takes no responsibility for her words or the effect they have. She simple pulls the words out of air, words that linger, waiting to be heard. Mercury knows it's up to the hearer to hear the words. Mercury's words are a balm to soften the heart hardened by hatred or to lighten the heart heavy with grief. If the balm is left on the nightside table, unused, forgotten, misplaced, ignored, Mercury shrugs her shoulders and carries on. There is always another message.

Let me tell you a story about Mercury and a message she offered a dying man who needed help to pass over with grace.

I was working night shift in a hospice for the dying. Working nights meant I spent the majority of my shifts talking with people who were dying. Mostly we talked about this and that, grandchildren and gardens, dogs and cats, favourite recipes and memories of childhood. Mostly, we talked to pass the time, as the time it takes to die is uncertain.

Sometimes though, we talked about the unfinished business from the life that was passing. Then I heard stories of unrequited love, regrets of frittering away life with meaninglessness, opportunities lost and words unspoken. Once I heard the confession of a murder. But this is a story about Dave. Dave told me one night that he was an asshole and he was afraid to die.

Dave was 52 and dying of pancreatic cancer. His body was skeletal, thin skin stretched over long bones. He was very tall. His lips were always dry, and he frequently sipped water through a straw as we talked to keep his mouth moist to wash away the bitter taste of his words.

The doctors had given Dave two weeks to live. Pancreatic cancer is usually a painful way to die. Most who die of pancreatic cancer spend their last few weeks doped up on morphine or fentanyl. Dave's cancer did not arrive with physical pain. While Dave was weak from malnutrition, his mind was clear. One night, he invited me to sit down and chat. He asked me if I believed in the Virgin Mary and the stories of her mercy. "Of course," I said wondering where this conversation was going to go.

Dave went on to say he had never gone to church and did not consider himself a religious person, but he had always had a good feeling about Mary. He asked if I knew anything about her.

I told him that I did not go to church either and did not consider myself religious. But I had faith in Mary. And I told him this story.

I was eighteen, just out of high school, when I accepted a job as an au pair in Paris. I thought of myself as adventurous at the time. I dreamt of being a writer. I thought every writer needed to live in Paris, sit in cafés drinking strong coffee and smoke cigarettes, while passing nights with a bottle of Bordeaux and a manual typewriter. Or, experience a ravishing romance, (the soul of poetry), and the style of a Paris nightclub. I was so naive.

The day I left for Paris at the airport I found a beautiful amulet of Mary, inlaid with mother of pearl. It laid at my feet as I stood in line to board the plane. On the plane, I hung the amulet on the gold chain I wore.

Mary traveled with me throughout that turbulent year. We walked the streets of Paris, Amsterdam, Barcelona and Geneva together. A year later and a little bit wiser, as I passed through customs at the Toronto airport, I reached to touch the amulet and it was gone.

Dave asked me, "Do you think she helped you at that time?"

"I am still here," I nodded.

Then he told me he had been an asshole, his word, to anyone who tried to love him. He wanted to know if Mary would help him make amends before he died.

"Of course," I assured him.

"How would I do that?" he asked.

I explained to Dave that prayer can be like a conversation. "Just talk to Mary out loud and explain to her the help you need. Tell Mary why you want her help. Be sincere." I offered to bring him a picture of Mary to help focus his mind while he talked with her.

He liked this idea and the next night I brought Dave a picture of Mary.

I was off work for the next few days and when I returned to the hospice Dave was happy to see me. With the help of his sister, he had made a list of the people he had been an asshole toward. His sister was asking each person to come and see Dave before he died.

There were 15 people on the list. As Dave expected to die in 10 days, he planned on two apologies a day. On the last two days of his life, he would rest quietly in his newfound grace and let death take him peacefully.

One by one his visitors arrived, uncertain, hopeful and looking slightly squeamish. His ex-wife paused at the nursing stations to ask if he was in pain. His stepson's girlfriend waited outside of his room, chewing her lip. His neighbour brought flowers from her garden. His former boss came straight from work, still wearing his uniform. As his brother-in-law walked by the nursing station he said he was only doing this for his wife. My co-workers and I watched the procession wondering what was going to happen.

We had worked around death for long enough to know nothing ever went according to plan. Death is after all the crossing of a surface and Mercury is the guide.

The ten days went by and Dave had made peace with his sworn enemies. He felt the grace of an unforeseen happy ending. Dave was ready to die a happy man.

Dave did not die. One day past the deadline, he asked me if he looked like he would die soon. I shrugged my shoulders, "Death comes when death comes."

Two days past the deadline, he was still sitting up in bed and getting a bit anxious. Three days after his due date and he was feeling better than he had felt in months.

First his ex-wife visited. "He must be lonely," she told us. She had brought a book of photographs from when they were married. "We'll remember the good times," she said. And into his room she went.

Ten minutes later she stormed past the nursing station, her mouth set in a tight straight line.

Next his neighbour showed up with more flowers. She left minutes later, leaving the flowers at the nursing station muttering something about that skinny bastard.

His boss showed up with a couple of the other guys from Dave's former work. They were in and out in record time.

That night Dave bitterly complained that Mary had tricked him. He had agreed to apologize to them but had never said anything about being nice. "I should be dead," was all he had to say.

The next day, his sister put up a sign on his door, NO VISITORS. And so, Dave was left to stew in his rancour for 6 more weeks before death arrived.

Mercury is tricky and makes no deals. Death is an all or nothing kind of event, as is healing.

Now you may be thinking, it was the Virgin Mary Dave had called on not Mercury. One must not be too literal when traveling across surfaces, as one never knows what will be found on the other side. All crossings are chaperoned by Mercury, and Mercury can take any form. She is the shape- shifter.

Dave had asked for guidance to cross over. This is Mercury's job. Mercury guides souls to their next destination after death. Dave asked the Virgin Mary, the great female healer who brings mercy to harden hearts, confused minds and lost souls, to help him seek forgiveness from those whom he had wronged. Whether the Virgin drew on Mercury's trickster energy, or Mercury wore the guise of the Virgin, I do not know. What I do know is Dave was not given a "Get out of jail free card." He was tested, and he failed. Dave's inner asshole could only be released by kindness to those he had harmed. Simple words would not do. Unfortunately, Dave did not appreciate Mary's message and died an embittered man.

Long, long ago, people believed birds guided the soul of the dead to the lands of the ancestors. Approximately 30,000 years ago someone carved a water bird, small enough to fit in the palm of the hand, its wings folded in preparation to dive from the clear blue sky into the ocean's deep cold waters.

Archeologists unearthed this bird, carved from mammoth bone, in a cave in southern Germany. They hypothesize this bird is the first human representation of the belief in Mercury's power to travel beyond surfaces and guide souls across the greatest boundary of all, life and death.

Thirty thousand years ago the unearthed bird, a gentle and fierce talisman was held in a Mercurial shaman hand as she penetrated life's ordinariness and plunged below the surface to the sea, flew beyond the vast starry night and descended into dark passages winding deep into the Earth, leading the souls of her people to their next destination.

Birds are hollow-boned creatures that defy gravity's pull and follow Earth's invisible magnetic fields across clear blue skies. Birds soar, glide, swoop through the sky in ways humans can only dream.

Each morning, bird song vibrates crisp spring air announcing Earth's turning to the Sun. Each evening their song announces Earth's turning toward darkness. Birds come and go, flit about and watch from treetops, speaking a language mysterious to the human ear. They are farsighted. Most birds easily take to the ethereal sky while some flow just as effortlessly between air, earth and water.

Birds are ruled by Mercury. Birds not only carry the gift of piercing surfaces but like Mercury, they are known for carrying messages. Old wives tell us that a bird in the house is a foreboding of death, black birds bring good news while being followed by a bird announces the presence of a guardian protector. Everyone knows spotting a robin is a sign of spring's arrival. At one time the art of augury, reading the flight pattern of birds, was practiced to understand life's big questions.

Through time Mercury has not lost his love of flight. Both the Greek and Roman Gods representing Mercury wore wings on sandals and helmet. Long before the Romans and the Greeks, the Egyptians gave their Mercurial god, Thoth, feathers. Thoth was one of the first Egyptian Gods to appear in their vast pantheon. Thoth had the body of a man and the head of an ibis, the water bird of wisdom.

Thoth gained his wisdom while standing next to Osiris, the Egyptian God of the Underworld, while he weighed the hearts of the recently dead. Hearts as light as a feather moved on to the next passage of death, a trial by 42 Gods. Hearts heavier than a feather were fed to the Ammit, a creature part hippopotamus, part lion, with the head of a crocodile, and were never seen again.

Thoth was the impartial scribe who faithfully recorded the good, the bad and the ugly found in the hearts of men. Seeing all that was contained in the hearts of men, Thoth became the ruler over chaos and order. Those who suffered from the unpredictable, hazardous and often unjust nature of life turned to Thoth seeking guidance on how to right a wrong.

When their hearts were heavy and death

approached, Egyptians petitioned Thoth for guidance in unburdening their hearts. Thoth offered the dying a safe place to rest before judgement. Thoth offered magic spells to overcome their troubles. While Thoth's messages mercifully provided the knowledge of how to die with a heart as light as a feather, it was up to the petitioner to lighten their load before meeting Osiris and his scale.

Thoth was a God of mercy, not judgement. Thoth was willing to show any heart, no matter how hard or heavy, the path to redemption. Few in our modern day consider Mercury to be as merciful as Thoth. Perhaps this is because we are short term thinkers and prefer to disregard the complex web just below the surface of consciousness that binds us to life.

There are small miracles in every life. Like the day when your car keys are misplaced and all your plans are ruined. As you cook dinner that evening, listening to the news, you learn that a tractor trailer rolled over on the highway you had planned to travel. If the day had gone according to plan, it is likely you would have met the truck moments before the crash.

Then there are curious life-changing synchronicities, like the time your friend cancelled a coffee date at the last minute and you struck up a conversation with a man at the next table. The man later became your husband. What about the time you acted on the feeling that you needed to call a friend just as they had fallen down the stairs and desperately needed help?

Mercury, while his messages are not always welcomed or heard, still offers mercy and an opportunity to right a wrong. The choice is yours on how you respond. You may blame Mercury for your interrupted plans, or consider the delay within the bigger scheme of things.

Mercury's plant Mandrake, also known as Mandragon, is like that—good or bad depending on how it is viewed.

The Egyptians revered Mandragon. Images of the holy plant are found adorning Egyptian tombs, coffins, mummy masks, temple and palace walls, cosmetic spoons and shards of pottery. The Pharaoh Tutankhamun was entombed wearing a necklace threaded with eleven Mandragon fruit. Osiris at times is painted wearing a crown adorned with ripe Mandragon fruit.

It's hard to know exactly how the Egyptians used Mandragon. There is no record of it in their Materia Medica compiled by Thoth in about 16 BC. Because Mandragon fruit holds a shape likened to the curve of a young woman's breast and was painted on the walls of tombs, temples and palaces, it is suspected that the Egyptians used Mandragon in both fertility and death rites reserved for royalty. A description of the following painting supports this theory.

> The small limestone relief Berlin AM 1500, which is known as "the stroll in the garden", shows a queen offering two mandrake fruits and a lotus bud to a king. The queen's gesture seems to suggest, in a metaphorical way, an initiation to sexual contact. Through the act of giving and the object given (the

> mandrake fruit), this iconographic scene may communicate a hidden message, that of the sexual contact which consequently implies renewal and regeneration: indeed, it is the queen who has to assure the continuity of the royal lineage through her body and fertility. (Casini. 2018).

TODAY, CHEMISTS SHAKE THEIR HEADS WHEN TRYING to understand why the ancients offered Mandragon as an aphrodisiac to enhance fertility. Its chemical constituents are more likely to cause a stupor than an erection. Perhaps it was not heightened libido the Egyptians sought when the Royal couple took Mandragon before sex. With careful dosing, Mandragon removes all inhibitions and opens up experiences beyond the surfaces of this world. As the high continues, Mandragon offers sleep rich in dreams that can last for days. Mandragon carried the royal couple out of this world and into the world of the Gods.

Beyond the superficial understanding of sex as a momentary release, those with some wisdom, like the Egyptians perhaps, understood the road of sexual pleasure is a dead end. The French refer to orgasm as La Petite Morte (the little death). It is said that transcendence of worldly desires and profound experiences of the divine are easiest to access during orgasm and at the moment of death. It is through sex that new life enters the world. The ancient Egyptians believed that it was not only sex that led to new life, but also death.

In numerous tombs, the Egyptians painted groups of women passing among themselves Mandragon fruit. The women appear to be smelling the fruit. It is speculated that the women were using Mandragon to communicate with the dead. Or perhaps they were taking part in death/rebirth ceremonies. It is hard to say several thousands of years later. One thing is certain, the ancient Egyptians clearly offered Mandragon a place within their death/rebirth ceremonies both as a psychotropic herb to use during sex and as a plant to guide their nobility through the Underworld to rebirth.

Mandragon more than any other plant represents Mercury as the guide through the Underworld. Mandragon offers Thoth's mercy to souls of the dying. A journey to Jerusalem during Roman occupation is necessary to fully understand this.

The Roman's had an infatuation for Mandragon. It was a favoured plant at their orgasmic parties that as time and emperors passed, crossed the line into the macabre. After sipping wine steeped in Mandragon, Romans released their inhibitions and crossed boundaries that today are considered cruel and horrific. Mandragon carried many royal Romans into the territory of madness. The boon many Romans saw in sipping wine imbued with Mandragon was that they not only lost their inhabitations and morality, but they also forgot themselves.

After taking a potion containing Mandragon, it was not uncommon for a Roman to wake up two days after a night at the emperor's palace and not recall a single thing about what had passed. Roman debauchery took place without guilt or shame. No matter what happened, one could carry on with a heart light as a feather.

Mandragon was more than a Roman party plant. It was an important part of their Materia Medica. They used it during surgeries as an anesthetic. Mandragon contains an array of alkaloids that act on the nervous system. The alkaloids atropine and hyoscyamine induce otherworldly visions and are the source of the journeys to the dark corners of the mind. The alkaloids scopolamine (which causes amnesia) and scopine weaken nerve signals to the muscles and this causes paralysis. This property was useful for Roman surgeons. It is easier to operate on a body if it is lying still.

The effects the plant has on the nervous system depends on the dose of the herb. A few drops of Mandragon numbs the pain of surgeries and amputations. Increase the dose slightly and Mandragon arrives with hallucinations of heaven or hell. Increase the dose again and the anatomic nervous system is significantly depressed. Heart rate slows. Lungs cease to expand and contract. Muscles are paralysed. At this point, Mandragon can bring death, or create the appearance of death. A little more Mandragon and there is no return from the Underworld.

The Romans made use of Mandragon medicine during crucifixions. The sentence of crucifixion was handed out for over 500 years. Being nailed to a cross was punishment for slaves, disgraced soldiers (read indentured labourers), foreigners and Christians. Crucifixion was not a sentence of death; it was a sentence of suffering. If you were lucky death occurred within six hours. Many hung on a cross for four days before death arrived.

The guards who watched over the cross-covered hills overlooking villages and towns occupied by Rome had a problem. They could not leave a prisoner on the crucifix undead. They were only given leave to return home after all the crucified were dead, taken down and tossed onto a pile of bodies. To speed up death's arrival, so they could go home, the guards stabbed and maimed the crucified. When that was not enough to bring on death, they offered them sips of vinegar, the best solvent for extracting alkaloids from plants, infused with Mandragon and Myrrh. Once the criminal was limp on the cross, like a dead man, he was taken down, tossed onto a pile of bodies and the guards went home to dinner.

It is easy to imagine Christ on the cross, suffering, Mary Magdalene weeping, begging the guards for mercy on behalf of her beloved. Did the guards, eager for the comfort of home, the arms of their wives and mundane stories of everyday life, a balm of ordinariness after a day of torture and murder, shrug their shoulders and wet Christ's lips with Mandragon's mercy?

I imagine Osiris and Thoth standing over the heap of maimed bodies on the hill overlooking Jerusalem, weighing the hearts of the dead against a feather. I imagine those with a light heart, waking to this world as Mandragon's medicine wore off, while others with a burdened heart journeyed more deeply into the Underworld. I imagine Mary with the other women gathering up Christ's limp body and taking him to a cave for burial, a burial that changed the course of human history when Christ transcended death.

Mercury is the messenger of the Gods. He is the healer's planet. Healers are messengers. It is not theirs to decide another's fate. No one knows when death arrives on the wings of Mercury or what the journey across the great divide will bring. For now, we live on surfaces.

VENUS, CAULDRONS, AND VERVAIN

Lucy is an ancestor of ours who 3.2 million years enjoyed sunlight's warmth and water's soothing caress. Named after the Beatles song "Lucy in the Sky with Diamonds", she was just over a meter tall and weighed about 28kg. She was the first to stand up right. This meant that not only did her pelvis tilt in such a way that she walked upright but she was able to gaze upon her lover's face the moment he entered her.

Before Lucy, there was only sex on all fours.

Imagine the first time our ancestor, Lucy an Australopithecus afarensis, orgasmed and fell into the light streaming from her lover's eyes. This was the moment sex transcended reproductive necessity and became intimate pleasure. This was the moment Australopithecus awakened to the ecstatic pleasure of entwining legs and arms and vagina embracing penis. When the Australopithecus faced her lover, she roused the rapturous energy of Venus every woman carries.

Ah, Venus. Beautiful, sensual, intimate and charming. Sex kittens purring and voluptuous bunnies seductively bouncing. And there is much more to Venus. My friend Charlene Jones, in her poem Passion Seed, expresses Venusian pleasure this way.

All, all animal, birds, plants, fish, insects
all seeing and hearing their way to each other
in hurly-burley motion
until all you know in all directions
is the latest clap of orgasm
shuddering across a planet
so used to ecstasy, so accustomed to climax
she throws it away in every detail free
as she continuously comes
tumbling between gravity and centrifugal force
this passion in space. (Jones. 1996).

VENUS IS MORE THAN SEX THOUGH. SHE IS THE mysterious synchronistic intelligence that guides life into being. Venus weaves the threads of harmony and beauty into the web of life. Venus brings to life vast and complex symbiotic relationships. The energy of Venus is woven into the synergistic relationship between plants and animals— plants release of oxygen essential to animal life and animals release of carbon dioxide plants need for life.

Venus' love of reciprocal relationships is found in the creeping web of mycelium, fine white threads of fungi in the first few layers of soil on the forest floor, exchanging nutrients with plants and providing defence against intruding bacteria and viruses. Venus is the play between trees, clouds, rain, lakes and the glass of water you sip. Venus is the Sun warming the air, stirring a wind carrying the scent of the milkweed to the monarch butterfly who seeks the plant where she lays her eggs. Venus hums in every cells of our being as mitochondria, a bacterial intelligence, sparks the energy of life. Venus is the endless web of symbiotic relationships.

Like networks of mycelium just below the leaf litter of the forest floor nourishing and supporting the life of trees and plants, Venus is Nature's intelligence weaving just below the surface of our linear mind with all its plans to seek order in the perceived chaos of life. Venus seeds the odd synchronicities, the unusual hunches, and the strange daydreams that seem so illogical at the time but become the germinal ideas birthing new life. Venus is the web of life. Venus is an invisible organizing intelligence creating beauty, harmony, pleasure and ecstasy for anyone who cares to pause in her garden for a moment.

If plants as a whole have a single ruling planet, I say it is Venus. As Nature's harmonious intelligence, it makes sense Venus rules plants. Plants nourish soil, cool hot air, calm winds, and call rain. Plants feed, house and clothe every living being on the plant. Plants make medicine, clean up pollution and heal our greatest griefs and deepest resentments with beauty.

Venus is the harmony that is always present in chaos.

Let me tell you a very old story about harmony and chaos from the Celts called The Cauldron of Change. I fell in love with Mara Freeman's version of the story. I have adapted it somewhat. If you want to read the original you can find it on her website Chalice Centre.

At a time when River sang lullabies and Tree told very long stories, there was a woman named Ceridwen. Ceridwen had two children, a boy and a girl. The girl was called Criedwy, Dear One, and she was as fair as a May morning's apple tree blossoms. Ceridwen's son however was ugly, crooked and stupid as a block. His name, Avagddu, meant utter darkness. Ceridwen loved her misshaped son and longed to bring brightness into his life.

What you do not know about Ceridwen is, she carried powerful magic. So, with her heart wishing to give her son beauty, knowledge and light she plotted and planned, researched and studied all the magical ways to heal all that ailed her son. She decided on a potion called The Cauldron of Inspiration. Those who know the language of the Trees, the Druids, say three drops from the Cauldron of Inspiration bestow the knowledge of all things past, present and future.

Ceridwen spent several months studying the sacred books of the Druids to be sure she would miss not a single detail needed to brew her special potion. She made a list of the herbs needed for Cauldron. She discovered under which Moon to gather the herbs and under which stars to steep them. She memorized the songs to sing over the brew as it boiled and knew when to stir the Cauldron clockwise and when to turn it counterclockwise. When at last she had gathered all the knowledge and ingredients together, she sang the ancient songs as she mixed the herbs with seawater in her great Cauldron. Finally she had to cook the decoction for a year and a day to make the charm firm and good.

Ceridwen was busy. She was a working mom with two young children. She did not have time to sit and stir the Cauldron all day and night for a year and a day. Nor did she want to wander the woods in search of twigs and logs to keep its fire from going out. Like any modern woman does with too much to do and not enough time, she hired a boy from a nearby village, Little Gwion to tend to the cauldron.

When the Sun shone, when the Moon rose and when the rain veiled the sky, Gwion stirred and stirred the simmering brew with a great wooden spoon. Every day he wandered the woods in search twigs and logs to keep the fire under the Cauldron hot. Its fire warmed his small body through the dark nights' chill. The scent of its herbs infused his mind with dreams. The song of its quiet simmer danced lightly in his heart.

When Sun rose on the day that the brew was ready, Gwion stirred the potion one last time, three times clockwise for good luck. Suddenly, three drops sprang from the Cauldron onto his thumb. The potion burned. Without thinking, Gwion sucked his red-hot thumb and swallowed three drops from the Cauldron of Inspiration.

In that very moment a great light filled his entire being and his young mind burst open. Everything that had ever happened and was going to happen in the world rolled out before him and infinity made a home in his heart.

But with his outer eye Gwion spied Ceridwen. Her face exploding with rage, she charged Little Gwion. The boy dropped the wooden spoon and ran.

Ceridwen in her madness was swift and was soon close behind the boy. Her footsteps thundered on the path. Her murderous eye pierced the flesh on his back. The boy ran and ran, and in his thoughts, he became Hare leaping to safety – and he turned into Hare and leaped away. Ceridwen turned into a Greyhound, and Hare was quick but Greyhound was quicker and soon Hare could feel Greyhound's breath on his neck. He bounded to the edge of the lake and leapt into the water. Gwion just then imagined becoming a fish, and Salmon he became swimming away through the dark reedy waters of the lake.

Ceridwen, using all her magic, leapt into the lake and transformed into Otter. Though Salmon was quick, Otter was quicker and just as her paws flexed to kill, Salmon leapt out of the water and in Gwion's wishes, became a bird. The boy became Crow and flew away. But as Ceridwen leapt from the water she turned into Hawk. Crow was quick but Hawk was quicker and swooped down and dug her claws into Crow's neck. At the last moment, Gwion turned into a grain of wheat and fell from the cruel grip of Hawk's talons onto the threshing-floor of a mill. And there Gwion hid with a thousand other grains of wheat.

Ceridwen did not give up. She turned into Black Hen and fluttered onto the threshing-floor. She scratched and pecked until she found the one grain of wheat she sought among many and swallowed it up.

No sooner had Black Hen swallowed the grain of wheat than the great cauldron rocked and swayed over the fire and with a great crack split in two. Black liquid oozed from the cauldron, dowsing the fire, and trickling away in a black stream poisoning all the land and all the horses grazing there.

In Ceridwen's belly the little grain of wheat began to grow. It grew and grew, and three months passed, and six months passed, and she was getting bigger and bigger and when nine months passed, she squatted down, grabbed the bough of a tree for support and gave birth to a baby boy.

Now Ceridwen knew who the baby was, and had continued to carry malice towards Gwion in her heart. As soon as the baby was born, she took a dagger and was about to slit the infant's throat when she accidentally glanced upon the baby's face. He was so beautiful. He was her own son. Ceridwen could not kill him.

Ceridwen threw the dagger down with tears of grief and frustration. Quickly she swaddled the babe in hides and laced him to a small reed boat. She tucked him under her arm and strode over mountain and meadow to the ocean. She tossed the little reed boat into the cold, salty water where it was tossed by the waves and currents for many hundreds of years. Strangely, the child did not age during all that time.

One May Eve day, a Welsh good-for-nothing, gambling, impoverished prince named Elphin decided to try his luck fishing for Salmon at the mouth of the

Conway River. He stretched his nets across the estuary and all night long he waited there under the bright stars. In the morning he waded into the water to see what he had caught. There was not a single fish in his net, but there was a wee boat all encrusted with limpets and barnacles. Within the boat there was something wrapped in many layers of animal skins.

Elphin folded back the skins one by one, and when the last one slipped off, there lay a little baby smiling up at him. Around the infant's head shone a bright light. Elphin could not believe his eyes. All he could say was, "Look at that shining brow!" And that is what he called the baby, Taliesin.

Taliesin became the Celtic Shaman Poet. After he had grown, he would write:

I was in many shapes before I was released:
I was a slender, enchanted sword...
I was raindrops in the air, I was stars' beam;
I was a word in letters, I was a book on origin;
I was lanterns of light for a year and a half;
I was a bridge that stretched over sixty estuaries,
I was a path, I was an eagle, I was a little boat on the seas.

(Freeman. 2021).

THERE ARE SO MANY LAYERS TO THIS STORY. LIKE ALL great stories, this story is a wise teacher. For now, we are going to focus on what this story reveals about Venus.

Ceridwen is a woman who carries magic. Magic is a kind of faith. Magic is the ability to let go into the moment and watch what happens. There is a saying that the greatest magician goes with the way the wind blows, not against it. The greatest magician understands the power of Venus – remember Venus is the mysterious synchronistic intelligence that guides life into being.

Nature is the magic the magician spins. Watching her son struggle, Ceridwen lost faith in Nature's magic. Desperate to make her son different from what he was, Ceridwen turned to manipulation and control of nature. Ceridwen's preference for light, and her distaste for darkness sent her down the path of managing, dealing with and handling the challenges she faced in accepting her son's limitations.

Anyone who gardens knows there will always be weeds, the ugly plants, and there will always be roses, the beautiful ones. This is the way of nature, the way of the world, the way of life. Discovering the medicine in the weeds and the medicine in the roses is the way of the magic.

The names of the six herbs Ceridwen gathered to brew the Cauldron of Inspiration are lost in mists of time. Many sources agree on four of them: Rowan Berries ruled by the Moon, Lesser Celandine ruled by Mars, Flixweed (*Descurainia sophia*) ruled by Saturn and Vervain ruled by Venus. The plant we are interested in here is Vervain.

In my garden Vervain grows taller every year. It is acclimatizing itself to the soil. In the garden Vervain has a gangly weedy look.

Vervain growing wild in a damp meadow takes my breath away. In the wild, Vervain is elegant. There is nothing weedy about it. Perhaps it is wild Vervain's graceful sway in the warm summer's breeze. Or the glimmers of light its tiny purple flowers catch twinkling in a sea of green. Maybe it is the plants' tall elegance that calls me closer. Vervain in the wild is enchanting. Some even call Vervain the Enchanter's Herb.

Throughout the land of the Celts, Vervain is a talisman worn to protect against any kind of evil, ill will or mischief. Taken with yarrow and eyebright, Vervain is used to treat *poc sidhe* (Fairy Stroke): a sudden and mysterious decline in one's mental or physical health.

Vervain carries much physical medicine, including supporting liver detoxification, rebalancing the sympathetic and parasympathetic nervous system and creating harmony for a woman's hormonal cycles. But it's Vervain's less tangible medicine that vibrates with the energy Venus.

Vervain's magic inspires a heart with compassion and opens your awareness to nature's beauty and abundance. In your heart, Vervain ignites joy and all the ways of love: friendship, partnership and family. Vervain helps you look within to resolve conflicts and understand how your innate goodness brings magic to the world.

Vervain is the herb of Inspiration and it is easy to understand why the Druids choose it for the Cauldron of Inspiration.

Let's for a moment imagine how Ceridwen's heart felt as she watched her son struggle through the simple things in life that another child delights in and masters with ease. Imagine her teaching him to hold a spoon, her hand gently wrapped around his, carefully guiding it to his month, praying he learns to feed himself. Imagine the difficult thought, "what will happen to him when I am gone?" The fearful thought is like a spider in her heart spinning a thick, tangled web of despair.

Culpeper writes of Vervain medicine in this way, "It warms up cold griefs in the heart." (Culpeper. 1992).

Ceridwen's grief must have been cold. Vervain, carrying Venus' medicine, warms the heart opening it to beauty. Did Ceridwen see the light in her son's eyes when she greeted him in the morning? Lifting him from his bed, did she feel the delicious warmth of his skin? Did she welcome his smile with her own? Even in the greatest darkness there is a glimmer of beauty. Venus ensures this. This is the medicine Venus brings to Vervain. Beauty is the medicine that warms cold grief.

And when we are no longer inspired by beauty, our lives turn to drudgery.

I love how herbalist Matthew Wood so succinctly named Vervain's medicine. It is for people who live by their lists. Or in other words, Vervain's medicine is for those who have lost touch with the intricate magical web weaving life into being. Vervain connects us with Nature's web, inspire us with the beauty of its intricacies and ignites creativity. Creativity brings wishes to fruition. Remember at the end of the story, Ceridwen received her wish; not the way she planned but nevertheless she had a son who is the best of all of us. Vervain, energized with Venus, brought Ceridwen's wish of inspired beauty to her cauldron.

This is how Venus' magical web of nature is woven: a

series of events that seem to always be going in the opposite direction but somehow spiral into fulfillment of our deepest heart wish (just not how we planned it). Or put another way, Venus grants our wishes, but often wraps it in gift paper we don't appreciate.

It is hard for a list maker to relax into Venus' web and let things work out the way they will. Over time, list making takes on a compulsive need to handle everything. Before you know it, the list trumps everything else in life. List makers have to stay focused, busy, accomplishing tasks, because if they pause, even for a moment, they will feel a shivering chill in their heart: the loss of faith in magic.

Pushing down the grief in the heart, list makers' days and nights become orientated around a never-ending to do list. Their relationships become focused on to-do lists. Even having sex gets put on a list. Their lives becomes lists.

I have never seen an inspired list. Lists lack spontaneity. For example, after a gentle rain a walk in the garden becomes a list of weeds that must be pulled. The moment to pause and imagine the bees snuggled in their hive waiting for the Sun to come out while lady mantel is embracing a drop of water shining like a jewel is lost. As is the moment when the list maker's heart rises to the wonder of nature's beauty and complexity, and all the worry life brings dissolves. This is Venus medicine; this is Vervain's medicine.

It is not surprising we would cover up our griefs with lists. Our culture is obsessed with lists and counting, accomplishments and forward movement. Take a simple social media marketing course and you are taught to catch people's attention with statements like: The Top Seven Herbs to Overcome Obsessive List Making, or Five Ways to Embrace Your Inner Venus, or Three Moves Guaranteed to Bring You to Orgasm.

Perhaps this is where Ceridwen lost control over the Cauldron of Inspiration. I bet she was a list maker. Her list was too long and tending to the Cauldron all day long, stirring it with the song in her heart and keeping its fire burning warm was written at the bottom of the list. She hired someone else to make her medicine.

Only you can make your medicine. I don't mean tinctures, teas, salves, etc. I mean the medicine in your heart, the medicine of inspiration, medicine carrying wisdom. Only you can create medicine that weaves your awareness into Nature's web, the medicine that allows you to rest in nature's paradox: everything is in chaos and everything is okay - Venus' medicine.

Ceridwen may have benefited from sipping a cup of Vervain tea to align herself with the great magic of Mother Nature before she set out on her great adventure with the Cauldron of Inspiration. Vervain's intelligence settles down the plotting, planning, preparing and doing. Vervain takes the managing, dealing and handling out of your hands. Vervain medicine brings a moment of pause, when you can sit in Mother Nature's garden and enjoy the beauty of life's cycles.

Would the story have turned out differently if Ceridwen had given herself over to stirring the medicine day and night? Would darkness have become light? Perhaps not. Nature's order is: darkness follows light and light follows darkness, just as Venus rises in the morning and she rises in the evening and sometimes disappears from sight. Venus is comfortable bringing in the light of day and bringing in the darkness of night. And sometimes doing neither. I suspect Gwion was always Nature's choice.

There are many meanings to the transformations Gwion and Ceridwen go through. One of the meanings the Cauldron's brew inspires is: when in complete union with Nature's web, anything is possible. Magic is spontaneous. In other words, throw away the plan, scrap the goals, tear up the lists. Magic is in the spontaneous moment when the heart opens to the beauty that is present. This is the true magic of Vervain and Venus.

After birthing the beautiful child, Ceridwen finds a good heart, and does not kill him (thank the Goddess), but tosses him in the ocean to be cradled by waves, rocked by currents and sung the many songs of water. This seems cruel and unusual, particularly from a patriarchal point of view, where only a birth mother can raise her child. There is a belief that only a mother understands her child's need.

In matriarchal cultures this is not how children are raised. Children belong to the community. It is the community's responsibility to feed, clothe, nurture, educate and love the child. Perhaps some part of Ceridwen, even though she carried great magic, knew this special child of hers needed something greater than she could give him on her own, so she released him to the Great Mother, Ocean.

> In the beginning....was a very female sea. For two-and-a-half billion years on earth, all life-forms floated in a womb-like environment of the planetary ocean – nourished and protected by its fluid chemicals, rocked by the lunar-tidal rhythms. Charles Darwin believed the menstrual cycle originated here, organically echoing the moon-pulse of the sea. And, because this longest period of life's time on earth was dominated by marine forms reproducing parthenogenetically, he concluded that the female principle was primordial. In the beginning, life did not gestate with the body of any creature, but within the ocean womb containing all organic life. There were no specialized sex organs; rather, a generalized female existence reproduced itself with the female body of the sea. (Sjoo and Moore. pg 2. 1987).

It's not surprising the Great Sex Goddess synonymous with Venus, Aphrodite was born from sea foam. The hot sexy wetness you feel between your legs when Venus calls for pleasure harks back to the great watery primordial erotic chaos once contained by Earth's vast Ocean.

The Greeks bestowed rulership of the ocean to Poseidon. To gain that power, the story goes, Poseidon abducted the Goddess Amphitrite, the ancient ruler of the sea, and made her his wife. The Greeks paid her small tribute, perhaps naming a boat or two after her.

In one Greek story Amphitrite reappears after her

abduction at the birth of Apollo, the Sun god ruling light, music and poetry, healing and plagues, prophecy and knowledge, order and beauty. Amphitrite moaned and swayed as the young god was birthed. Amphitrite is the waters of the sea and the waters of the womb.

Vervain knows how to support a woman in labour. While commonly referred to as a uterine stimulant, I think of Vervain as more of a uterine synchronizer. During birth the uterus pulses like ocean's waves. The contractions rise and fall, contract and relax. When waves of birthing rise and fall, sway and moan, in a synchronized rhythm, birth is easier. Vervain brings harmony to the ancient waves coursing through uterus, the woman's body and the child about to be born.

Recalling the story of Apollo's birth, one cannot help but think of Taliesin. Taliesin with his shining brow was rocked by the ocean. Ocean, The Great Mother, infused the helpless babe with the knowledge of all that has been, is and will be. She bestowed upon him the gifts of poetry and healing. Gestating in the womb of the Great Mother, washed over by her many moods and whispered her endless stories, Taliesin learned plenty. As do all beloved sons in their mother's wombs.

Seawater is a favoured solvent among witches. Ceridwen chose it for brewing the Cauldron of Inspirations. Circe, the magnificent witch from Greek mythology, used seawater in her potions of transformation. Seawater, the birth place of the ecstatic chaos of life, is an essential ingredient for anything magical, like the birth of a child.

It wasn't until Age of Reptiles, approximately 200 million years ago, that the first penis attached to an amphibian slithered out of the ocean and onto land. That is not that long ago considering Ocean first tossed and turned like a restless lover over Earth 3.8 million years ago. It took her a long time to birth penis. Penis remains a force of Nature that continually seeks the ancient waters found in the womb cave, that penetrating force that stirs a woman's cauldron 'til sheets are drenched with salty sweat, the force that plants the seed in the waters of wombs.

And so we return to sex and our ancestor Australopithecus turning for the first time to face her lover, guiding his penis with her hand to her vagina as they fall into the light of each other's eyes forever changing the way we love. This is the power of Venus.

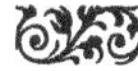

VENUS, DIRT, AND VIOLETS

When Botticelli painted Venus as Aphrodite, she was sweet with loveliness, her gaze was tender and her nakedness was innocent. He imagined her coasting on a colossal scallop shell, luminous as a pearl, gently blown by a warm breeze to the shore. Roses floated on the air greeting her. On shore the Goddess of Spring waited for her with silken robes delicately embroidered with clusters of plants.

Botticelli's painting of Venus evokes feelings of beauty and blessings. It is a celebration of naive love. Botticelli's painting is as serene as the calm before the storm.

The Babylonians describe their Venus, the Goddess Inanna, as having breasts like storm clouds. Her loving fertility tumbled across the sky with thunder. Her passion ignited bolts of lightning, defying darkening skies. The fury of her storms sent the bravest man and woman racing to shut their windows, lock their doors and cower by fire, praying her ripping winds and slashing rain would leave them whole.

Anyone who has ever been blessed by Venus, fallen head over heels in love, knows it is not all grace, beauty and harmony. There is aching loneliness, raging jealously, unquenchable desire, cruel words and the many morning afters when hurtful silence is broken with tears of remorse.

Venus has many faces—the morning star which ushers in the light of day and the evening star which brings in the dark of night. For 263 days Venus shines as the morning star in a sapphire blue sky as morning light swallows night's darkness. Then the planet's light disappears into the bright blue of daytime skies for 50 days. Venus then shines for 263 nights on the edge of the horizon as twilight falls.

Venus appears on the edge between waking and sleep, morning and night, conscious and unconscious. Venus nudges us towards the edges of distinct realities like light and dark, dream and awake, and asks us to travel along the blurred lines of liminal spaces where rigid beliefs become unbearable and change is demanded. It is Venus, with her uncertainty, beauty and ugliness, harmony and discord that compels us to surrender and fall into the grace woven into the web of life.

Life brings many edgy moments that offer opportunity to embed ourselves within Venus' grace. Moments on the edge are difficult though. At these liminal moments in life words are lost, beliefs shaken, identity stripped away and we are humbled. Let me tell you about one of these moments in my life.

I was in school studying to become an herbalist and working part time in a hospice caring for the dying. For many years death had fascinated me. Now that I am older, I do not feel the same intensity to understand it as I did when I was younger. These days death becomes more of an inevitability. When I was younger, I thought about death a lot and I was drawn to work with the dying in an effort to understand this great mystery. After caring for one particular woman, death no longer pulled on me. The morning after her death, as Venus rose in the sky, I woke up with Lucinda Williams singing in my head, "I am learning how to live."

I cannot even recall her name now. It was a simple name, something like Ann or perhaps Carol. I will call her Ann. She was probably about as old as I am now, maybe a little younger. I do recall her grandson, a babe in the arms of her daughter-in-law. I was trying to get pregnant at the time, and I remember stroking his soft cheeks with a longing in my heart.

Ann had been transferred to the hospice in the night and was there in the morning when I came on shift. The night nurses reported she had been heavily sedated for the transfer and was still sleeping. We were told Ann had breast cancer with metastasis to the spine and brain. My care-partner and I shifted uncomfortably in our chairs at the thought of the tumours in the spine. Unrestrained growth in the spine creates pain that is difficult to control. This meant moving Ann would be difficult no matter how careful we were.

The tumour in her brain could mean anything. Once we had cared for a woman with a brain tumour whose hunger ravished her. She spent her last days eating anything she could get her hands on, donuts, apples, hamburgers, popcorn, salad. The brain tumour in another patient caused his arms and feet to continuously flay about. The poor man was exhausted by the unceasing, uncontrollable movement. Another brain tumour caused a man's speech to come and go. To this day, I can remember his incredible sense of humour about it all. We had no idea what the brain tumour meant for Ann and her final days.

My partner and I, even though we had experience caring for those with breast cancer and its metastasis, were not prepared for what we found when we went into Ann's room to "freshen her up" for the day. Removing her gown and the dressing from her breasts, we were confronted with ulcerations covering her entire chest. Where her breasts had once been was now weeping, red sores that smelled of rotting flesh. The sight of her breasts and the odour completely overwhelmed us. Everything we had ever felt about our bodies at that moment changed.

A long, long time ago, Venus, as the Goddess Inanna, was turned into rotting flesh. But I am getting ahead of myself. Let's begin with who Inanna was.

Inanna, the Babylonian Goddess called The Queen of Heaven, was beautiful, rich and powerful. Anything Inanna wanted she was given. All she had to do was ask. Inanna was famous for her sexual appetite. No man could turn her down. And when a lover bored her, she cast him aside discourteously.

Inanna's story is the story of a woman who was addicted to sex as power. It tells the tale of a woman's fall from grace. It is about what happens when a woman forgets to surrender to the harmony and beauty of Venus' complex web of relationships. Inanna forgot how to listen to her intuition, empathize with the pain of another and let things be. The story of Inanna is about a woman deeply identified with an idealized image of the body coming to terms with the earthly nature of flesh.

Recently I was in a circle of women and I asked them what they thought of when I said the word Venus. One woman replied, "Shaving my legs, like that ad for razors. You know the one by Bananarama, 'I'm your Venus, I'm your fire, and your desire.'"

When sexual desire is determined by the amount of hair on a woman's legs, Venus' inherent pleasure that ripples through flesh becomes distorted. When shaving the hair off your legs is likened to casting a spell over a man's desire, sex becomes a power game not the dance of pleasure.

When a woman uses her sexuality for power and not pleasure, Venus too becomes sick. Sex as power often holds hands with sex as commerce. Sex in exchange for protection, shelter, food, or perhaps jewels, fine wine and status, is not sex as a physical expression of love and pleasure. When a woman uses the gifts of Venus for commerce and power her body morphs into an object. She becomes a sexual object. All of her beauty is pushed aside as her Venus, her feminine intuition and grace, is sexualized. Not that sex is not part of Venus' embrace, but it is so much more. There is an intelligence to sex that becomes lost when the body is objectified.

Inanna's story begins when she meets Gilgamesh, a great warrior hero whose fame, like wildfire was spreading far and wide as he returned from war triumphant. Inanna was drawn to Gilgamesh like a moth to a flame. She needed to bathe in the glow of his fame and conquer his desire and body. She wanted him on her leash. Inanna plotted and planned, whispered in ears her desire and soon she was sitting next to him at a great banquet held in his honour. She invited him to her bed.

Gilgamesh had nothing but scorn for the likes of Inanna. He turned to her and said so all could hear,

> Your lovers have found you like a brazier which smoulders in the cold, a backdoor which keeps out neither squall of wind nor storm, a castle which crushes the garrison, pitch that blackens the bearer, a water skin that chafes the carrier. (Mark. 2011).

Gilgamesh's insults turned Inanna's world upside down. Before him, her every wish had been granted. She had wanted for nothing. She had not known the feeling of a desire unfulfilled or longing for fulfillment. She did not know the hope for difficulties and misfortunes to end. Inanna felt entitled to have her desire fulfilled as quickly as possible, no matter who was hurt, humiliated or pushed aside. Inanna's sense of entitlement made her heartless. She had not suffered as lesser beings do. There was no suffering to spark compassion in her heart.

Gilgamesh and his slight awakened new feelings in Inanna. It was untenable to her that she could be rejected. Casting aside the pain of rejection, Inanna raged and sought revenge. Revenge took Inanna to a very dark place.

Ann raged. She did not know why she suffered. The metastases that penetrated Ann's brain caused extreme disorientation. She did not understand where she was and who we were. Her confusion created fear. The fear turned to rage. She abused us with names like sluts and bitches. Throwing food. Hitting. Kicking. Exhausted by the extreme emotions, Ann wept and finally slept only to wake and go through it all over again.

Horrified and helpless, her family watched. "She was always such a kind person," they would say eyes pleading for understanding. "She is a good Christian woman so how can this be?"

As Ann deteriorated mentally, the cancerous ulcers covering her breasts began to ooze puss and the smell of rot filled her room.

Caring for Ann was hard. We dreaded her rage and the stench of the cancer eating her breasts. The charcoal pads we folded into the dressing over her breast and the air purifier did nothing to ease the nausea we felt entering the room.

But that was not the worst of it. We were witnessing

the dehumanization a disease could bring to any woman. It was immediately apparent to us that the tortured woman we tried to care for could be anyone of us. My partner said many times upon entering Ann's room, "But for the grace of God go I." Ann's breasts were our breasts. Ann's flesh was our flesh. Ann's mortality became our mortality. Ann's descent was acutely felt by all those who cared for her.

Innana's rage triggered her descent from Queen of the Heaven to rotting meat hanging on a peg in the underworld. Her descent began when in her rage she demanded her sister's husband battle Gilgamesh. Gilgamesh butchered him.

Once more humiliated Inanna retreated, remorseless until the sounds of her sister's weeping seeped into her awareness like a sliver under her skin. Eventually she had to visit her sister to make amends.

Inanna's sister was Ereshkigal, The Goddess of the Great Below, Goddess of the Dead. Ereshkigal had been birthed from sorrow. It is said Sky, heart-broken, wept when he was separated from Earth. And when the Sky God's tears mixed with the salty waters of Earth's ocean, Ereshkigal was born. Later, as those born from sorrow often are, Ereshkigal was separated from her family by a dragon who raped her and dragged her into the Underworld. Once in the underworld, Ereshkigal was forsaken by her family. Having mingled with the dead, she was now unclean.

There were many women with breast cancer who came to the hospice to die. Some were young mothers whose death broke our hearts. Others were old women of whom after they passed, we whispered, "Perhaps it is for the best." But we had never seen suffering like the suffering Ann was subject to. The torment of her mind and the humiliation of her decaying breasts was more than anyone should bear. It was too much for her family. They stopped coming to see her.

"She isn't my mother," her son wept.

Babylonian history tells us they believed there are seven gates which a soul passes through on its way to the Great Below. At each gate, pieces of identity must fall away. And so it was for Inanna. At each gate, she lost something of her power, something of her status, something of her beauty, until she stood naked, bowing before her sister, her horrible, unclean sister riddled with grief from the death of her husband. Inanna was responsible for this death. Ereshkigal fixed her with a look:

> She fastened her eyes upon her (Inanna), the eyes of death,
> Spoke the word against her, the word of wrath,
> Uttered the cry against her, the cry of guilt,
> Struck her, turned her into a corpse.
> The corpse was hung from a nail.(Brinton-Perere. 1981).

THE ORIGINAL TELLER OF INANNA'S DESCENT GOES ON to describe the smell of Inanna's rotting flesh hanging from a post.

I was not working when Ann died. At the hospice when death arrived peacefully we used the euphemism, "It was a good death." When death did not arrive with peace, we avoided each other's eyes saying just enough to let it be known death had been unkind. Ann's death was like that. Her spine had snapped as the nurses turned her. So many slip away in silence. Ann died with her eyes open, writhing in pain like a worm on a hook.

Shortly after Ann's death I was working on my plant monographs for school. I had 300 or so to do that year. A plant monograph is a basic outline of a plant's medicine, its actions, chemical constituents, indications, traditional uses and so on. I was researching the medicine Violet carries preparing to write its monograph, when I came across the following passages in Bartram's Encyclopedia of Herbal Medicine:

> (Violet) Has a long traditional reputation as a mild analgesic for cancer of the lungs, alimentary tract and breast (poultice). When the wife of General Booth, Salvation Army Chief, was dying of cancer the one drink that gave her relief from the pain was Violet leaf tea made from leaves foraged from railway embankments by devoted members of the Army.
>
> Lady Margaret Marsham, 67, was cured of a malignant tumour in the throat with Violet leaf tea taken freely. Compresses of the leaves were also applied, with immediate relief from pain and breathing difficulties. Within 7 days the swelling disappeared, within 14 days the tonsil growth as well (Bartram. 1998).

"As if!" I thought in disbelief as I read these passages, "I have seen cancerous ulcers." I was not prepared to believe that a poultice of Violet leaves could heal the rotting ulcerations that were once Ann's breasts.

Most who journey to Ereshkigal's realm do not return. It is the realm of the dead after all. But like Venus returning after disappearing from view for 50 days, Inanna's flesh was redeemed with life and she returned to her place in heaven to shine.

Inanna's faithful servant pleaded for her mistress's case before the god Enki, whom the Greeks later named Mercury. Enki, like Mercury, does not follow rules and is endlessly creative.

For reasons of his own, Enki felt mercy for Inanna and from the dirt under his finger nails he formed two small creatures called the Gala. The Gala passed into the Great Below, like flies, and found their way to Ereshkigal.

What you do not yet know about Ereshkigal is she was pregnant at the time of her husband's death. When Inanna arrived in the Great Below, Ereshkigal was about to go into labour. When the Gala arrived, she was in labour, "No linen was spread over her body/ Her breasts were uncovered/Her hair swirled around her head like leeches." (Brinton-Perere. 1981).

The Gala, seeing Ereshkigal's misery, pain and aloneness sat down beside her and offered her their acceptance.

Being made of dirt, the Gala had no pretenses, nothing to hide and no knowledge to give. All they could do was acknowledge and accept Ereshkigal's as she was. They moaned as she moaned. They cried out when she cried out. They raged as she raged. They shared her suffering.

After reading the piece in Bartram's about the Violets, hot vulnerable feelings rose up inside me. The claims that Violets could have eased Ann's suffering felt crass and insincere. This made me angry. I went for a walk.

It was spring. A chickadee followed me flitting amongst the aspens' luminous green leaves, chirping its happiness. As the path turned, I came upon Violets, a ribbon of delicate purple flowers cradled in heart-shaped leaves. They were tiny plants growing close to the earth reaching for a touch of sunlight. Standing amongst the sweet beauty of the Violets my heart opened and I wept. I wept for Ann, her family, my colleagues and myself. The tears carried the frozen lump of fear from my throat and the hot rage of injustice from my heart.

Ereshkigal must have wept when she heard the Gala moan with her pain. For in the end, she gave them the medicine they needed to renew Inanna's flesh. Revived, Inanna returned to her place in the heavens rising as Venus does after a period of absence.

Inanna was a Goddess ruled by her passions. She cared little for the hearts of others. She sought only her own gratification. When Gilgamesh spurned her, it is said she killed hundreds with no regret. It was the burning intensity of her passion that paved the way to her sister's realm of the dead.

Ereshkigal was a Goddess also ruled by her passions. When Inanna entered her sister's realm, with a single look Ereshkigal turned the supreme Goddess of the Heavens to meat. That was passionate hatred.

It was the cooling medicine of dirt that saved both Goddesses from their passions. Have you ever sat under a tree after working in the garden on a hot July afternoon? Feeling flushed with heat, your hair damp with sweat, the earth cool in the shadows of the tree draws heat from your body. You emerge refreshed of body and mind. Heat will always move towards coolness. This is the second law of thermodynamics.

Violets ruled by Venus carry moist, cooling medicine that gently pulls heat from tissues, cooling not only inflammation in the body but also the inflammations in the mind. Venus, of soft curves and loving whispers, offers medicine that softens hard views and beliefs that keep us from the change that the blurry lines of liminal spaces offer.

So it is with a poultice of Violets. Violets, particularly their leaves, carry medicine called mucilage. It is this medicine made from complex sweet sugars, that cools the heat of inflammation. Even if a poultice made with Violet leaves does not appease cancer's hunger, it will momentarily ease the intensity of its burn. I wish I had known this for Ann. Easing pain in the body will often bring some comfort to the mind.

Sometimes I get really lucky and someone gives me a tincture they made with all their love. This happened last summer with a tincture of fresh Violet, flowers and leaves. There are no other words to describe the feeling this sweet medicine gives me but comfort. It makes my heart serene.

There is not much written about how Inanna's journey to the Great Below transformed her. Perhaps she became a more compassionate Goddess, I do not know. But I do know the journey I took with Ann changed me. Witnessing her suffering brought me to my knees, humbled me.

Violet, the flower quick to bloom and quick to die, reminds us that in the end there is only our being human. The word 'human' comes from the word humus, or dirt. As does the word humble. Violets, like dirt under fingernails, are a symbol of gentle humility. The lowly-growing Violet shows us how we can rise and fall and rise again through the humility taught when we surrender to the beauty of life.

MARS, LUST, AND NETTLES

Albrecht Altdorfer was the first European renaissance painter to bring to life wild landscapes with dark forests, fiery suns and haunting twilights devoid of people. In Altdorfer's landscape paintings people did not cut down trees, hunt great stags or till the land. Altdorfer, like other painters from his time, also painted Bible stories. One of the paintings Altdorfer is most famous for is the biblical story Susanna and the Stoning of the Elders. Susanna was a favoured subject of painters during the Renaissance. Susanna was painted over and over throughout the time of light, as the Renaissance is referred to. If I had to choose the portrait of Susanna I preferred, I would choose Altdorfer's.

Susanna's story comes to us from the Hebrew Bible. Susanna was a beautiful woman with a good heart. At a young age she married Joakim, a wealthy man who was a leader in his community. Her husband owned a large house where he conducted his business and community affairs. It was not unusual for the house to be filled with businessmen as well as senior Court Elders who gave advice on affairs of the community, and laid judgement on those who had done wrong.

To get away from the busyness of her home, Susanna, with her maids, walked every day in the orchard behind her husband's house. There she enjoyed the stillness and beauty of nature while contemplating the presence of God in all of life.

Susanna's beauty caught the eyes of two senior court Elders and they fell into a state of lust for her. Every afternoon as she walked in the orchard, the two men, hidden even from each other, tracked her through the grand old trees and garden like hungry dogs, pawing and sniffing.

One day each caught the other spying on Susanna and it was then they hatched a plan to fulfill their lust.

It was a warm day. Susanna had decided to bathe while in the orchard. She had sent her maids to gather her perfumes, oils and clothes. As soon as Susanna was alone, the Elders sprang on her, demanding she lie with them. When she refused, they threatened her with an accusation of adultery before the courts which, of course, they controlled. The penalty for adultery was death by stoning.

Frightened and desperate, Susanna cried out. Hearing her calls for help, her husband, the businessmen and the court officials rushed out to the orchard to find Susanna half-dressed. Standing by were the two court Elders who, pointing their long shameless fingers at Susanna, told the men they had seen Susanna with a young man. Susanna was sentenced to death by stoning. It was an open and shut case.

As Susanna was led to her death, a young man stepped forward named Daniel. He questioned the Elders and soon it was clear that they were telling lies. Susanna was set free and the Elders were stoned.

Renaissance painters portrayed Susanna's suffering many, many times. During the Renaissance, the church forbade representations of a woman's naked body. Susanna is one of the few women in the Bible who could be painted naked while being true to a biblical story. Perhaps the Renaissance painters portrayed Susanna to fulfill their need for freedom of expression. The female body is beautiful and has been the muse for many great artists. But a quick survey of the many paintings of Susanna during that time suggests otherwise.

Few painters were as kind to Susanna as Albrecht Altdorfer. In Altdorfer's painting the two Elders are seen crouching behind a patch of Nettles as they plot, plan and leer. The Nettles in Altdorfer's painting carry ambivalent meaning. During the Renaissance, Nettles was taken to improve a man's sexual force. It was a lustful herb. By the same token women of the time used Nettles for protection.

Nettles is a prickly plant and incites a stinging rash if handled recklessly. One of the first places I ever saw Nettles growing was in a back alley in the east side of Vancouver, in a neighbourhood where teenagers are often seen on street corners exchanging their sneakers for stilettos. Someone had planted Nettles along their fence to keep these young and uninvited guests out. Nettles were seen as easier to care for than a big dog with a nasty bite.

One word often used to describe the energy of Mars is anger. As an expression of speech, to nettle someone is to annoy, irritate and anger. Anger, like Nettles, can form a protective barrier around a woman. No one wants to mess with a bitch. Every woman, although Mars is considered male energy, carries the vibration of Mars. Every woman has the capacity to use anger to form a protective barrier around her. During the Renaissance women created protective barriers by using Nettles.

Did Albrecht place the nettles between Susanna and the Elders for her protection or as a sign of the Elders' lust? I suspect Albrecht added the Nettles to the painting for Susanna's protection.

At the time that Albrecht painted Susanna, the courts were beginning to find women guilty of bizarre actions liked crazed orgies involving animals and eating children. Over the next two hundred years women were hunted and tortured. It is estimated that 100,000 women were put to death by fire, water and the rope. Women were tracked by witch hunters, men following the guidance of church and state. The same men who offered the witch hunters guidance, oversaw the humiliating trials the women endured. As the hunting intensified so did the sufferings of Susanna.

In 1580 an unknown Flemish painter portrayed the Elders leering over Susanna, their hands circling her naked body while she looks away, her eyes dark pools empty of light.

In 1607 Flemish painter Peter Paul Rubin created at least 5 paintings of Susanna. In one of his paintings the Elders approach Susanna from behind and grab the cloth she wraps herself in, revealing her nakedness. Susanna looks back at the Elders with fear and confusion.

In 1622, English painter Anthony Van Dyck paints Susanna with eyes flashing wild with fear while one of the elders pinches the flesh on her upper arm as if testing it for texture and plumpness.

By 1647, Dutch painter Rembrandt Harmenszoon van Rijn paints the elders pulling at Susanna's clothing as she collapses into herself and turns to the viewer with pleading eyes.

Did Altdorfer foresee the torture and murder of women during the Renaissance? Was he warning women to be careful of the court officials hunting them and intending harm? By placing Nettles between Susanna and the Elders was he telling women to protect themselves?

The Renaissance was a 300 year period that spawned many of Europe's greatest thinkers, authors and statesmen. It was a time of rebirth following the long shadow of death cast over Europe during the terrible plague years. Renaissance men guided Europe from darkness to light while science replaced superstition. The Renaissance provided an environment for men to thrive. Women, however, did not fare so well.

The Renaissance was driven by the energy of Mars.

It was a time that burned with a creative, passionate fire fuelling the lust to rise again from the ashes of the plagues. Renaissance men were determined to move forward at all costs. Consumed by the flames of renewal, many of these great thinkers and statesmen did not see the darkness left behind after the fires had gone out.

Francis Bacon (1561-1626) was an English Renaissance man. He was a prolific writer of poetry, science fiction, (before it was a genre,) and several influential treatises on Natural Philosophy. Each piece of Bacon's writing envisioned a bright future for mankind, one of discovery, knowledge and wealth. Today Bacon is called the Father of Empiricism and the Inductive Method used for scientific inquiry. This is sometimes referred to as the Baconian method, or simply the Scientific Method.

Bacon also led an active political life. Trained in law, he climbed the ladder to the highest position in England, the Attorney General of England.

Lastly, he was a religious man, as most men were during his time. Historians believe it was Bacon who encouraged his boss, King James I to sponsor a new translation of the Bible while Bacon himself oversaw the work. Further, it was Bacon King James chose to write the opening dedication of his new Bible, the King James version now most widely used.

King James is said to have been a stupid, crass man, if cunning and forceful. He was also a witch hunter. Before becoming King of England, James was King of Scotland where he encouraged the burning of 4,000 women over a 14 year period and wrote a treatise on how to discover, question and punish a witch. This treatise was called Daemonologie,

> The fearfull abounding at this time in the countrie, of these detestable slaves of the Devil, the Witches or enchanters....that such assaults of Satan are most certainly practised, that the instrument thereof merit most severely to be punished. (James. 1597).

BACON ALSO WROTE OF WITCHES, "THE OINTMENT that witches use, is reported to be made of the fat of children digged out of their graves; of the juices of smallage, wolf-bane, and cinque foil, mingled with the meal of fine wheat." (Lee. 1627).

In overseeing the translation of the King James Bible, Bacon ensured that any reference to a witch be feminized.

While men of science continue to praise Bacon for his remarkable understanding of inductive reasoning, feminist historians and eco-feminists are not so kind to him.

Eco-feminist Maggie Rose Berke writes of Bacon:

> I do attempt to bring to the attention of environmental scientists, that our discipline is gendered at its core, with its forefather, Francis Bacon, being the chief employer of violent gendered language, encouraged by experience with the witch

hunts to shape an exploitative and industrially useful theory of nature.(Berke. 2017).

WHILE SUPPORTING HIS BOSS' NEED TO HUNT DOWN and murder women, Bacon was writing his revered work on how to dominate nature through scientific inquiry in order to enrich the lives of men. He wrote these treatises using the language of the witch hunts, trials and murders and likened Nature to a woman's body.

He encouraged science in "hounding nature in her wanderings, to be able to lead her afterwards" (Bacon, 1980, p. 72-73) and advised men that "the secrets of nature betray themselves more readily when tormented". (Bacon, 1620, p. 268). He used the language of rape as another method of investigation, "penetrate beyond proper means of decorum." (Bacon, 1620, p. 262-263).

He told his readers that nature (always using feminine pronouns) and all her creatures have no will of their own, "for the whole world works together in the service of man...Plants and animals of all kinds are made to furnish him...insomuch that all things seem to be going about man's business and not their own." (Bacon, 1609, p. 747).

Eco-feminists even suggest that a study of the Maleus Malificarum (The Hammer of the Witches) a "book designed to be a thorough dissection and diagnosis of what makes a witch, how to identify behaviours of witches, and how to correctly prosecute them"

(Kramer and Sprenger 1486) and second in sales only to the Bible between 1487 and 1669, influenced Bacon's organizing principals of Scientific Method.

Eco-feminists suggest that if during the time of Renaissance women had not been hunted down, their bodies not probed, poked and pricked in search for the mark of the Devil and then hung, burnt or drowned, and the leading scientific minds of the time like Francis Bacon had not referred to nature or viewed nature as a woman's body needing to be dominated, we would not be living in our current state of ecological devastation. Eco-feminists draw a direct line from the burning times to our current environmental crisis.

But we all know women and nature have not fared well since the burning times and history is written by the victors. Mars, like the Renaissance men, insists on winning at all cost. What does this have to do with Nettles?

Let's unbury the history of women hidden in the light of the Renaissance and see how Nettles and Mars fit in.

Nettles is a very common plant. It grows close to humans. Often when a plant grows close to humans, herbalists say it offers friendly medicine. This means that one may use it with little fear of side effects or harm. Friendly plants are good for everyone.

There is an expression amongst herbalists, "When in doubt, offer Nettles." I don't agree with this off-the-cuff saying herbalists use. Nettles carries the energy of Mars and too much Mars can cause trouble. For instance, once I was speaking about women's health and mentioned Nettles. A woman spoke up and told me she was allergic to Nettles. This seemed very curious to me as it's not the kind of plant that causes allergies. Often Nettles is used to calm allergic reactions. After the talk, I asked the woman why she thinks is allergic to Nettles.

She told me she was drinking Nettle tea to increase breast milk. This is reasonable as Nettles does increase the nourishment in breast milk. One of the principals of Mars is supporting strong growth.

After a few weeks of drinking 3 cups a day she developed terrible stomach pains and could not eat anything. She stopped drinking the Nettle tea and the pains went away. Even more curious now as I had never heard of Nettles having such a dramatic effect on a stomach, I asked the woman if I could see her tongue. The appearance of the tongue offers herbalists a glimpse into what is going on in the digestive system.

Her tongue was bright red, raw looking, and hard. This is a sign of too much heat in the body, specifically the digestive system. The vibration of Mars creates heat in a plant. Nettles, carrying the energy of Mars, was encouraging further heat in her digestive tract, making the imbalance in her body worse.

Long before the light overtook darkness, women spun thread and wove fabrics for clothing in their homes. Every article of clothing was made by a woman's hands. Women used different types of material to make their clothe. Wool and silk were preferred if a woman had status and privilege. Most women used what grew close to home. Nettles grew close to home and their stalks could be spun into a sturdy thread that made a tough but pliable fabric. Cloth made with Nettles can withstand strain and time.

Imagine it's a sticky afternoon. The air is thick with the scent of lilacs and roses. In the distance children howl with laughter as they plunge into river waters. Cicadas sing. In the cool shadows of a small stone house, a woman is humming soft words to the gentle thump of her spinning wheel. Beside the wheel are stalks of Nettles. She is spinning Nettle thread. Into the thread she chants "May iron not bite the one who wears this."

Or perhaps we can imagine this scene another way. As the children swim in the river, women are gathered in the shade of an oak tree. They spent the morning gathering nettle near the shores of the river. The leaves are now drying in baskets. The stalks lay next to their spinning wheels. The women are anxious and comfort each other. The church has called their sons to march to the Holy Land in a crusade against the infidels. Their sons are eager for heroics. The women do not need heroes for sons. They just want their boys to be alive and whole. As they spin Nettle into threads, they chant, "May iron not bite the one who wears this."

Before the Renaissance and burning times, women were the councillors in the village. They mended broken hearts, resolved conflicts in their communities, supported women in their birthing, helped the dying go gently and offered healing to everyone in between. They carried the plant knowledge of their Grandmother's Grandmother. They were taught the ancient rituals and words that bestowed blessings. They could foretell the weather, find a lost lamb and hear the wind's story of the time to come.

Simply put, women were responsible for the physical and spiritual well-being of their communities. They were very busy. They did not have time to walk to special places for prayer and guidance, nor did they have time to take time out of their day to pray and meditate. Their spiritual life and prayer were woven into their daily tasks. A favoured time for prayer was while a woman spun and wove cloth.

The gentle repetitive motions of spinning and weaving eases one into a naturally meditative state. The act of making clothing for their families was part of every women's spiritual discipline. Women before and during the Renaissance put their prayers into the fabrics they made.

The meditative focus and intention infused into Nettle thread as a woman spun her prayers offered the plant a magical aura. All those good intentions created the belief that Nettles protects people from ill wishes made by others. It was said Nettles had the power to break curses and ward off the evil eye. Women were known to carry and give away small swaths of Nettle cloth to shield the ones they loved.

This finely woven relationship between Nettles and women lasted for centuries, until the Renaissance and the movement away from the darkness of superstition and into the light of science.

The energy of Mars must have been so strong at that time. The bloodthirsty quest for power by the Church and State was brutal and vicious. These male dominated institutions were so threatened by a woman's power to spin her prayers into the threads she wove that they tortured and murdered between 100,000 and 9,000,000 women over a 300-year period. Clearly this is dark and irrational for the time of light and reason.

During the Renaissance, medicine moved from a woman's home and into the hands of men and monks in monasteries. Plant names, the names women had passed from one generation to the next, were Latinized. Latin was the language of the Church. Only those who spoke Latin had direct communication to God or could heal with God's blessing. The plant names the women healers had used for centuries were forgotten as one healer after another was convicted of witchcraft and murdered and names of the plants were changed.

When the court officials or clergy lead the women to their execution, whether by burning, drowning, and any number of horrible deaths, they dressed the women in homespun Nettle shirts. By doing this the Inquisitors believed the Nettle shirts protected them from any curse the woman threw towards them during her final moments on earth.

The belief that Nettles offers spiritual protection runs deep in the veins of human beings.

As I write this it is about a year since the Me Too Movement exploded on social media. The Me Too Movement brought voice to thousands of women who have faced sexual harassment and assault. A year ago, everyone began talking publicly about the dirty secret women have endured for a very long time.

Speaking out prior to Me Too, although many did,

was frightening and the consequences dire for most. A year after the voices of thousands of women rose, every day in my clinic I meet women and their anger. Anger that has been pushed down. Anger that has not had words. Anger that has been called to voice by the Me Too movement.

While social media offered a platform for the Me Too movement, there are many different opposing views posted daily. Like this one: *Karma is a bitch, only if you are!* This expression Nettles me. Sometimes, when the bitch, a woman's Mars energy, is suppressed, karma can take a brutal turn. Brutal for the woman, that is. The energy of Mars makes strong physical and energetic boundaries that will protect a woman and keep her from harm. Mars, while being challenging for most women taught from girlhood that a "bitch" like a "witch" is scorned or worse, creates confidence and a strong NO. Every woman needs a swatch of Nettle cloth in their pocket.

MARS, WOLVES, AND HOPS

I am standing outside in the snow. It is cold. Ice crystals form on loose strands of my hair that have escaped from my tuque. The others in line stomp their feet trying to stay warm. We are standing outside a small stone hut waiting to participate in a ritual that will initiate us into fierce compassion.

As I stand there in my mind's eye a wolf appears limping across the snowy field towards me. The wolf is bone thin and mangy. Her one eye is swollen closed. On her head she wears a crown. Glints of gold shine from under its dented tarnished surface. It hangs crooked on her head. The wolf is proud and tattered. She walks beside me as I enter the darkened room for the initiation.

The wolf is ruled by Mars. Mars' energy infuses the wolf with a furious appetite. Mars drives the wolf in its relentless hunt for the flesh of another. The wolf's aggression is attributed to Mars, the malefic planet, the planet of bad luck and obstacles. The wolf has come to symbolize the worst of Mars.

There is an old story called the Great Bound Wolf that comes to us from Norse mythology. It is the story about how a wolf came to embody the dark side of Mars.

A wolf named Fenris was born to the giantess whose name was "Sorrow-bringer." Some also called her the Great Mother Wolf. Fenris' father was the capricious shape-shifting God Loki. At Fenris' birth, it was prophesied that he would kill Odin while the entire cosmos came crashing down ending all life. This is a time the Norse called Ragnarok.

Odin is the Norse God who relentlessly sought wisdom for wisdom's sake. In old Norse his name means "Master of Ecstasy." He was the leader of the old Norse Gods. Many adventurous tales are told about him: the discovery of runes, giving up an eye in exchange for wisdom, hanging from the Great Yggdrasil Tree and stealing the Mead of Poetry from giants. Odin was a hearty-drinking mate who knew a few card tricks and a merciless warrior willing to spill blood for honour's sake. The Norse referred to him as The War-Father. A prophesy of his death struck fear in the minds of the Gods. Seeking to undermine the prophesy and ease their minds the Gods took Fenris as a pup under their care.

Fenris was an unusual pup, cleverer than most, with an enormous appetite. When he began to grow at an alarming rate the Gods became fearful. The fear awakened cruelty in their minds and they began to conspire against the wolf. They agreed something must be done to restrain his power. The Gods decided Fenris must be bound before he achieved his full strength.

The Gods tied a heavy metal chain to a sturdy pole and taunted Fenris, "You are not strong enough to break this chain."

Fenris examined the chain with a calculating eye and decided he could easily smash it. He agreed to be bound. As soon as the last link was fastened, with one mighty swipe of his razor-sharp claws, the chain shattered into pieces.

Concern mounted about the wolf's strength and the Gods renewed their plotting to bind mighty Fenris. Another chain was created, stronger and more durable than the first. Again, the Gods taunted Fenris. Again, they bound the great wolf. Again, in a single swipe of his massive paw, the chain shattered and Fenris was free.

The Gods were now terrified of Fenris' strength, intelligence and power. Swallowing their pride, they turned to dwarves to twist them a rope to bind the great wolf. The dwarves wove a rope with the magic of things that do not exist: the silence of a cat's footsteps, the beard of a woman, the roots of mountains, the breath of a fish, and the spittle of a bird. Once the spells had been cast, the dwarves presented the Gods with a rope as fine as a silk thread.

Once more the Gods called to Fenris and taunted him, "You are not strong enough to break this bond." They showed him the thread. Fenris sniffed the air and caught the scent of a trap. He considered his options, pacing up and down and shrewdly eyeing the Gods, he said:

> If you bind me so that I am unable to release myself, then you will be standing by in such a way that I should have to wait a long time before I get any help from you. I am reluctant to have this bond put on me. But rather than that you question my courage, let someone put his hand in my mouth as a pledge that this is done in good faith. (Faulkes, 1995.).

THE GODS SQUIRMED AND DELAYED UNTIL FINALLY the God of War, Tyr, agreed. He put his arm in the wolf's mouth.

When Fenris rose to swipe at the thread, it tightened, and his jaws snapped shut and he swallowed the God of War's hand.

Fenrir raged and roared. He shook with fury at being trapped. As Fenris let out an Earth shattering howl the Gods quickly pushed a sword into his open mouth. They jammed the hilt of the sword into his lower jaw while the blade's tip threatened to pierce the roof of his mouth. Fenrir's rage was silenced. A stream of foam infused with betrayal and revenge ran from his mouth forming a river later called Expectations.

Quickly the Gods knotted the thread through a boulder and there Fenris paced madly plotting his revenge at the end of world, Ragnarok.

I was deeply moved by this story when I read E.S.

Wynn's empathetic writings of Fenris, "Fenris is pain. Fenris is the tortured and bound wolf soul of Old Europe." (Wynn, 2020).

It has not been easy for wolves in Europe. The last wolf in England was killed in the early 1600's after King James I ordered three wolf hunts a year. One hunt occurred in the spring when the female wolves were nursing blind pups in their dens. The last wolf in Scotland was killed in 1684 and Ireland's wolves became extinct in the late 1700s. They disappeared from the watershed of the Rhine in 1899. In recent history, Sweden's last wolf was hunted and killed in the 1960s and in Norway the 1970s. It is not hard to imagine Fenris struggling to break free of his bounds and wreack his revenge across Europe on behalf of his kin.

It was hunger in Europe that ignited the war between humans and wolves. In 1315, a Little Ice Age crept over northern Europe shortening the growing season causing the Great Famine. Over a two-year period approximately a quarter of northern Europeans died of hunger. As if that was not enough, the Black Plague arrived in the mid 1300s, killing another third of the population. The wolves, also hungry and opportunistic, could not resist the easy prey of livestock. Imagine the outcry of the desperate people. They may not have been able to protect their families from hunger and the plague, but wolves, they were an easy target to set sights on, hunt down and kill.

Before the plague and before the famine, Europeans had a symbiotic relationship with wolves. Wolves were the guardians of crops. German folk lore tells about a number of spirit wolves who protected the small plots of cleared land tilled for growing grains within the great forests that covered northern Europe. There was the Roggenwolf (rye wolf), Getreidewolf (grain wolf), Kornwolf (cornwolf) and Gerstenwolf (barley wolf). E.S. Wynn suggests these wolf spirits who watched over a farmer's field were once real wolves. Wynn speculates that at one time farmers welcomed the presence of wolves. A nearby pack of wolves kept the deer from grazing on and wiping out their crops.

Mars not only rules appetites, anger and revenge, but also rules over agriculture. As a guardian of agriculture another side of Mars presents itself. Growing food is most productive when it is an organized community effort.

My friend Sami Shaman, Ailo Gaup (Gaup is the Sami word for wolf) told stories about wolves teaching humans how to live in community. He taught that each wolf in the pack has a role to play in the survival of the whole. Ailo emphasized the inherent understanding wolves have that as individuals they will not survive if any member of their pack goes hungry. The wolves instinctually manifest the fierce compassion of "no one is left behind". Every member of a wolf pack has value.

Biologists are fascinated by the wolves' communal behaviour. As a wolf pack travels through their territory, it is the older or sick wolves who lead the way. The slower wolves set the pace for the movement of the pack. This way the wolves do not leave behind or cause hardship for their slower member. However, if there is an ambush, these are the members of the pack that are sacrificed.

Following behind the old and the sick are stronger wolves. In the middle of the pack the younger wolves safely ramble and play as they cross the wilderness. Behind the pups there is another set of stronger more mature wolves. The wolf bringing up the back is the alpha. From this position she can see everything and control the movement of the pack through signals with her tail, facial expressions and sounds.

Considering the movement of wolves through a landscape, I am reminded of the ancient Romans, people whose ancestors were suckled by wolves. Rome's legionnaires marched across Europe, following their leader wrapped in a wolf skin. The wolf skin, a symbol of a fierce spirit, represented the Roman's carefully crafted military maneuvers and systematic process of implementing civil laws in order to conquer the tribes of old Europe.

The energy of Mars and wolves is complex. Both represent the basic survival instinct of life which turns to aggressiveness when threatened and can explode into homicidal rage. However, when left in peace with space and time to consider options, Mars and wolves both carry the cunning intelligence necessary to transform the instinctual life force into dynamic and corroborative systems that support the wellbeing of entire communities. A pack of wolves in the untamed wilderness with deer, beaver, squirrels and fish, keeps a distance between themselves and man knowing the human is the only predator more deadly than themselves. Confine the wolves' territory and limit their food supply and cattle and sheep become a dangerous food source wolves are willing to risk their lives for.

Was it the Gods' betrayal of the pup they had promised to raise that caused malice and revenge to twist Fenris' mind until he became completely mad with murderous rage? Was it the Gods' fear and their decision to bind Fenris that led to Odin's death? In the end, it was the hungry wolves lurking in the shadows of the Gods' minds that led to the Gods' demise.

In a psychological astrology chart a healthy Mars manifests as a dynamic creative will, capable of facing life challenges head on with confidence. The wolf manifests this will. Wolves are fearless. They move across the wilderness, an unsentimental instinctual energy, with grace, stealth and power.

If the creative will in a human is thwarted with oppressive institutional belief systems, limiting social economic status, or bad parenting, the dynamic will cowers like a chained animal while deep within rage smoulders. When silenced the fiercely compassionate creative energy of Mars retreats to the shadows of the psyche festering like a boil filled with pus waiting to burst with revenge. A creative dynamic will, like the wolf, needs to be able to run free.

Hops, a favoured plant of brewers, is ruled by Mars and named after the wolf. The plant's botanical name is Humulus lupus. In Latin Lupus means wolf.

Plants that carry Mars' signature tend to be warming or hot, like mustard and cayenne. Mars plants tend to be aggressive, demanding change within the body, forcing a healing response like inflammation. My Mom still shudders when she tells stories about my Grandmother's mustard packs on her chest as a kid and the blisters the packs left behind.

Some plants ruled by Mars offer gentle medicine like Hawthorn, a tonic for the heart. Hawthorn as a plant is fierce. Its long thorns are as sharp as wolves' teeth. When picking the shrubs' flowers or haws, pay attention for the thorns will pierce skin.

Herbalists of old probably gave Hops the rulership of Mars because it supports a glutenous appetite. The plant's namesake, the wolf, is able to eat twenty pounds of meat in one sitting. Hops eases the stomachache after gorging at all-you-can-eat buffets. Hops helps the body break down the deep-fried fats, sweet and sour chicken balls and ginger fried beef are saturated with.

After wolfing down her share of the meat, a wolf will curl up and have a good long sleep. After eating at an all-you-can-eat buffet, Hops lull you to sleep like a baby while your stomach digests the greasy food that without the herb would have caused heart burn, a grumbling gall bladder, painful bloating and insomnia.

Hops as medicine that eases indigestion caused by an insatiable appetite fits Mars' signature. However, Hops estrogenic effects contradict Mars' manliness. Hops frequently makes it ways into formulas for menopausal women relieving night sweats and insomnia while taking the edge off bitchy irritability.

Men who drink large amounts of hoppy beer, or work around Hops everyday suffer from a condition called "Brewer's Droop" and their chests blossom with

'Man Boobs'. Hops' estrogenic activity is contrary to Mars virility. Beer ads with buffed surfers, beefy line-backers and brawny lumber jacks are misleading.

In Europe there was a time when women were the brewers and recipes of fermented drinks with a kick of alcohol called gruit were passed from mother to daughter. Gruit is the mother of today's beer.

Gruit was a rich nutritional drink made with field and garden herbs like Nettles and Raspberry leaves. Some gruits were brewed for their medicinal properties using herbs like Birch leaf, Meadowsweet and Rosemary. Special gruits were brewed to celebrate seasonal rituals. These gruits contained dream herbs like Mugwort and Henbane.

Most women brewed gruit for their families. It was a liquid multi-vitamin during a time when fruit and vegetables were a rare treat. If a woman was a skilled brewer, she made money on the side, selling her gruit to neighbours, at markets or to a passing traveller seeking refreshment. Brewing was part of woman's income. This lasted until the introduction of Hops into the art of brewing, a plant ruled by Mars.

The problem with gruit was it had to be made every few days. Even though it was a fermented alcoholic drink, it turned sour quickly causing nausea and loose bowels. It wasn't until the 12thcentury that famed herbalist, musician and radical abbess, Hildegard of Bingen let slip in her pharmacopeia "Physica Sacra" the old monastic secret of Hops preservative power to the world of brewing. Hildegard's fellow Benedictines' had been adding Hops to their monastic brews for at least 2 centuries before Hildegard revealed their special ingredient.

It must have been a knowledgeable Benedictine herbalist who first added Hops to the daily beverage favoured by monks. Just think of all those men cloistered away behind high stone walls. A daily dose of an estrogen bearing plant would have been a welcome respite from testosterone's libido and go and get 'em approach to life.

Hildegard also warned the brewers that while using Hops in their fermented drinks would cut down on a woman's daily tasks, it would have unfortunate side effects. She warned that too much Hops causes melancholy to descend into the soul.

Melancholy or not, there was money to be made by adding Hops to gruits. Hops' preservative effects allowed the homemade nutritional drink to be produced in large batches and stored. Beer was born.

Over the next three hundred years, brewing was taken from the hands of women and industrialized. Seeking to monopolize profits from this favoured alcoholic drink, men only brewing guilds were formed and woman brewing in their home, with little income and no political power, were unable to keep up with the newer brewing methods. When a woman continued to brew beer, she was ridiculed as an "ale-wife" (ale being another word for gruit) or worse accused of consorting with demons.

In 1550, an English poet named John Skelton blathered a misogynistic poem about an alewife called The Tunning of Elynour Rummyng. The poem dehumanizes the ale wife with hideously vicious descriptions of her appearance, morals and brewing methods.

> Beginning by telling us that she is 'Droopy and drowsy/Scurvy and lousy', Skelton than details her features: her face bristles with hair; her lips drool 'like a ropy rain'; her crooked and hooked nose constantly drips; her skin is loose, her back bent, her eyes bleury, her hair grey, her joints swollen, her skin greasy. She is of course, old and fat. She is also ridiculous, wearing elaborate and bright clothes on holy days and cavorting lasciviously with her husband like – as she proudly tells it in Skelton's poem – 'two pigs in a sty'... (Bennett, 1991).

'RESPECTABLE WOMEN' NO LONGER MADE THE nourishing, medicinal or ceremonial gruit for their family and community. Women lost a portion of their independent incomes. By 1540, it had become illegal in some areas, such as the city of Chester, England, for women between the ages of 14 and 40 to sell ale.

Ale houses had been around for a while before the brewing guilds were formed. They were usually a family home where a woman lived who was a talented brewer. When Hops became a staple in beer production, independently standing ale houses sprang up everywhere. Twenty years after Skelton wrote his disgraceful description of an alewife there was one licensed ale house for every 187 people in England. In the ale houses women, unless they were willing to sell something other than ale, were not welcome.

Where once the farmer, the black smith and merchant would have been happy going home after working hard all day to enjoy a mug of his wife's gruit, now men went to drink in the alehouse, away from home, wife and family. In the alehouse they drank beer made with estrogenic Hops. This new drink did not enrich men with the power of local herbs brewed with their wives love. Instead Hops infused beer bound their spirited Mars virility to a thirst that could only be quenched in a room full of men drowning in their beer or worse, nursing their grudges.

The Egyptians understood the taming power of beer. They needed something beyond exhaustion and whips to bind the slaves that dragged the massive stones across the desert to build the pyramids. After reading this story about Ra, the Sun god and beer, I have to wonder if beer was not a link in the chain that bound the slaves.

Ra, the All-Powerful, was infuriated by the disrespect humans were showing him. He resented their lack of gratitude towards his creations. With punishment in his heart, Ra summoned Sekhmet, a furious Goddess in lion form.

"Kill them all," Ra demanded of her pointing at the humans below.

Sekhmet, purred and licked her lips. Bloodshed was her speciality. Ra watching from above feasted on Sekhmet's brutality as she tore the heart from every human who crossed her path and devoured their flesh.

The Earth became soaked in blood. When the cries of terror and grief reached Ra's ears, he became horrified by what he had done. He had to stop Sekhmet's rampage.

So he sent a great rain of red-coloured beer to the place where Sekhmet hunted. The beer was red because it was strained through pomegranates. The red beer ran down streets and soaked fields like huge pools of blood. When Sekhmet came upon these red pools, she paused to quench her thirst thinking it was blood. Soon Sekhmet stumbled and forgot Ra's orders and her rampage. Drunk, she curled up and went to sleep. When Sekhmet woke, she had been transformed into the peaceful Goddess Hathor, the cow goddess.

Sekhmet's connection to beer has been memorialized in an inscription found over her temple in Dendera, Egypt, "The mouth of a perfectly contented man is filled with beer."

In Europe the rise of the ale houses took place during a dark historic time. It was a time when fear seeped deep into women's hearts while men drinking pacifying hoppy beer were lulled to sleep like Sekhmet. It was the burning times.

I remember the first public talk I gave as an herbalist. Actually, I was a fourth-year student and had just completed my thesis, "Is There a Place for Herbal Medicine in Long Term Care?". I was presenting my thesis at a conference for nurses working in senior care. Just before I was to make my presentation, I gathered with the rest of the conference's participants to listen to the keynote speaker's address.

The first slide of his power point presentation was a cartoon of a woman with green skin, a long nose with a hairy wart at its tip and a pointy black hat. She was stirring a bubbling black pot with three legs, chanting "Boil and toil." The keynote speaker, a MD and PHD, began, "Those witches, ha ha, oh, excuse me, I mean herbalists are always brewing up some sort of misinformation."

The hair on the back of my neck stood up, my heart pounded in my chest and I froze in place. It was not until the room was empty that I got up and walked out.

In the 1500's, the height of the witch hunts, women and their cauldrons, the most common cooking pot in any household and one often passed from mother to daughter, were demonized. Their brews were called treacherous, diabolical and poisonous. Women who carried the knowledge of their grandmothers were publicly humiliated and murdered while recipes as old as time passing from matriarchal lineages were hidden and in time forgotten.

Shakespeare wrote his famous scene of the three witches, brewing up a treacherous spell. It reflects this time. The brew these malevolent spirits in women's form chanted over is still famously recited in most high school classrooms where English literature is taught—

IN THE CALDRON BOIL AND BAKE;
Eye of newt and toe of frog,
Wool of bat and tongue of dog,
Adder's fork and blind-worm's sting,
Lizard's leg and howlet's wing,

For a charm of powerful trouble,
Like a hell-broth boil and bubble. (Macbeth: IV.1 10-19).

Discussions of witch hunts, trials and murders during Shakespeare's time are not part of the curriculum. Shakespeare's portrayal of women brewing up evil mirrors the views of that time. It is unfortunate that no great man of letters wrote of the money jiggling in the pockets of the member of brewing guilds as husbands and fathers whiled away their time in Ale Houses spending household income on alcohol that at one time was freely made by their wives.

I have to wonder if male-only ale houses and brewers' guilds made the witch hunts possible. Where were the men I have to ask when their daughters, wives and mothers were being hunted down and burnt alive? Exhausted by manual labour and beaten down by life's uncertainty were they cowering in their pints of beer, their courage lost to a stupor? Were they bound to their thirst like Fenris was bound by magical thread of things that do not exist?

I picture the witch hunters, men paid by the brewers' guilds, arriving in a town. Discretely the witch hunters inquire after women who carry the knowledge of brewing while men sit in the Ale House drinking beer trying to quench the thirst of their never-ending struggle against poverty. From within the walls of the ale house, no man could muster the fierce compassion needed to protect his family from the grave danger the witch hunters brought to town.

Seen in this light Hops, a plant ruled by Mars, takes on the dark side of the red planet. It becomes a servant to the privileged few: the privilege of being the top dog in a dog-eat-dog world. Lurking within privilege there is always fear—fear of the loss of status, comfort, power. It is a fear that needs to bind those who create uncertainty. The fear often takes the face of one less fortunate: the dog beneath one's knee.

Mars' powerful vibration becomes distorted when focused on self-interest. Wolves know how to use the power of Mars. Wolves understand an individual only thrives when everyone eats, and no one is left behind. The alpha wolf does not hurt the weaker wolves who set the pace as the pack roams through the wilderness. He protects them with fierce compassion.

The wound caused by Fenris' binding, still bloody and raw, drove him to kill Odin. In the end Fenris died a villain, struck down by the sword of Odin's son.

The wolf, however much biologists teach us about their intelligence and collaborative ways, continues to be maligned. What child does not learn the implicit warnings contained within the fairy tales like Little Red Riding Hood? Don't trust the wolf or follow the path into the wilderness your creative spirit wishes you to take. Bind yourself to safety. No matter how it hurts, only follow the path of the way things have always been done. Drink beer and watch the football games. Whatever you do, don't fire up your cauldron and brew up some medicine.

JUPITER, DOORS, AND OAKS

If you sit in a quiet place beneath an aged Oak tree, your back supported by bark gnarled with time, and breathe gently into your heart letting the hopes and fears of days settle like still water, after a moment or two your ears will open to the wind's whisper through the leaves of the great tree. If you listen for a little while, you may hear the song of the future or perhaps a song from the past.

It is New Year's Day. Last night big sticky snowflakes fell from grey skies. This morning the forest is a magical wonderland of twinkling light. Tree trunks are decorated with tuffs of fluffy whiteness. Branches hang over the path draped with mounds of snow. Garlands of ice crystals sparkle on naked twigs. There is stillness and then a chickadee's song, short and sweet.

I gaze at the small grove of young Oaks that stand at the entrance to the deeper forest where I walk daily. The bark on their trunks is thin and smooth with youth. Their hopeful branches reach for the sky. My mind turns to the famous Oaks that once lined the path to Glastonbury Tor in Somerset, England. Somerset is where my maternal Grandmother was born.

There are just two Oak trees there now, on the path to the Tor. They are called Gog and Magog. Their hollowed trunks support limbs that twist like ancient arms embracing the sky above and reaching down to touch Earth below. If you gaze gently into the bark of these ancient one, faces with gentle smiles and painful grimaces begin to emerge. It's as if seasons past have been etched into the wood of these great trees. The Oaks, Gog and Magog, are named after the last two Giants to live on the isle of Britannia. Legends tell us that they were the only two to survive a bloody battle between the giants and the first King of England, Brutus. After his victory, Brutus dragged Gog and Magog to London where they lived out the rest of their lives in chains.

Beneath the young Oaks at the edge of the forest near my home, I wonder why my Great-Grandmother left Somerset to cross the ocean, a child in her womb while holding the hand of a two-year-old. A soft voice mingled with the wind sighs, "The old ways were dead; they were gone with the trees."

The year my Great-Grandmother left Somerset the procession of ancient Oaks that shaded the path leading to Glastonbury Tor were cut down. Farmland was needed. One of the trees was 2000 years old.

Long ago when stories and dreams were as real as you and I, the Tor was the sacred Isle of Avalon. Avalon was the magical land where apple trees' limbs hung heavy with fruit no matter the season and crops were always ripe with golden grain. It was a place that knew no hunger. Morgan the Fey, the great enchantress from the Arthurian legends, was Avalon's guardian. She spun the magic that nourished Earth's abundance. Morgan the Fey, often portrayed wearing a long flowing black cloak, her beauty shadowed by a wide hood, was the Brave King Arthur's sister and sometime lover, his mortal enemy and his healer. Rarely in the stories of men is Morgan the Fey the one who tends Earth's bounty. Often, she is degraded to a witch that meddled with Arthur's love life.

Long before the area around Somerset was drained to make way for agriculture, a great marsh covered the land. Here and there, throughout the vast stillness of the marsh, islands rose. These islands were strange places veiled in swirling mists rising from the silent marsh waters. The islands were shaped like the great mounds where the ancient Celts buried their dead. Or where, some say, dragons slept hoarding gold and jewels. One of these islands was Avalon.

It was through the marsh's twilight mists that Morgan the Fey rowed her small boat carrying King Arthur with his mortal wound. It was to the magic of Avalon that Morgan took the Great King to die. It is there he is buried. The prophesy Morgan left behind tells that when there is great need for a leader just and wise, Arthur will rise again.

I gaze at the young Oaks lining my path in the snowy wonderland. Their ochre leaves edged with soft white snow twirl as they cling to the branches reaching high in the sky. I guess the need for a leader, wise and just, has yet to be great. The icy grip of winter chills my heart. The past is so dark, as is the future. Seeking certainty is constant. Another voice rises on the wind, "Yes but the Oaks still grow, and they do not let go easily." A flame ignites in my heart.

The Celts, my Great-Grandmother's ancestors, loved Oak trees. The Oak was honoured for its generosity. Before the forests were cut down and the land plowed, the Oak's acorns were a staple in the Celts' diet. The Oak's hardwood offered fire and shelter. Oak bark provided the Celts with medicine to stop bleeding wounds and rid the body of poison. The Oak was the Celt's most sacred tree: gracious and benevolent. It was from the Oak they sought guidance. For the Oak grows so old, it knows there are no sins that cannot be forgiven. The Oak was the Celt's honoured ancestor.

The Celts believed they were descended from trees. To the Celts the forest was their vitality because all trees were their ancestors. They were not wrong. About 1.5 billion years ago human and tree DNA split. Today 15% of our DNA comes from trees.

Amongst the Celts there were men and women who trained for 20 years to learn the language of trees. These were the Druids, the councillors of the community. In Gaelic, the language of the Celts, Druid means the Knower of the Oak. The Gaelic word for Oak is duir. Duir means door.

Oak trees are ruled by Jupiter, the planet that brings a change of luck. All one needs to do is respond to the knock on the door and welcome in the unwelcome guest to profit from Jupiter's benevolence.

Jupiter is an enormous planet, the biggest in our solar system. Over fifteen hundred planets the size of Earth can fit inside its massive girth. Its brightness sparkles in the night sky. Only the Moon and Venus shine brighter.

Jupiter is Earth's protector. Astronomers call Jupiter the vacuum cleaner of the solar system. Its colossal size creates an extensive gravitational field that sucks into it all sorts of space debris, such as comets and asteroids, barrelling across the universe. Some of this debris, if left on its trajectory would slam into Earth. The great planet protects Earth from terrifying collisions with space debris.

Jupiter is Earth's shield.

Astrobiologists, people who study the possibility of life beyond Earth, speculate that space rocks ricocheted off Jupiter's gravitational field and were flung to Earth seeding life on this blue planet.

One could call Jupiter a doorkeeper for Earth. The planet keeps the unwanted space debris out, but allows the seeds of life in.

There is a very old story tucked in amongst the Arthurian Legends about the beneficence of the Oak tree and its role as a doorway to abundance. The story takes place while Arthur was still a young man. Like most young men, Arthur thought he had something to prove. He was at a stage in his life when setting an agenda and trumpeting his accomplishments were important. The robe of the Great King felt too big for his young body. The burden of the crown made him feel like an imposter. Arthur needed to prove himself. He did not yet understand that the beneficence of life does not come from the acts one makes in the world stage, but from the generosity of one's heart.

Because of his youth and lack of experience he was jealous of another great leader, Bran. Bran had ruled the Celts long before Arthur was a twinkle in his father's eye. Like Arthur would one day, Bran had united the Celts and reclaimed the land from invaders. The Celts deified Bran and buried his head under what would become Tower Hill in London.

It was common belief that as long as Bran's head was buried under Tower Hill, the land of the Celts would flourish. It was the reverence for Bran's head Arthur could not stand.

Unfortunately, by the time Arthur came along, once again the Celts were fighting off invaders, and coping with the frequent skirmishes that broke out amongst themselves. Some believed Celts were yet to be unified because Bran had made a fateful error during his reign. He had gifted the Great Cauldron of Annwn, The Cauldron of Plenty, to the Faery. The Faery are the forever young who dwell in the Twilight Land.

In the Celtic world The Cauldron of Annwn offered many gifts to whoever tended it. The cauldron granted poetic inspiration and prophetic knowledge. It fed and nourished all who asked for sustenance from it, other than cowards. The cauldron did not feed cowards. It favoured the brave.

Some renderings of this old story say that the Cauldron of Annwn revived soldiers who had died in battle. There was, however, a price for renewed life. There is always a price. A reborn soldier gave up his voice.

For a king like Arthur destined to unite the Celts and fight back invaders in the lands, a cauldron that renewed a fighting force would be a boon. Arthur thought that if he possessed the Cauldron of Annwn, the crown would feel more comfortable on his head.

So, Arthur set sail from Camelot to the Twilight Land with three ships carrying knights ready to die for his cause. It is said Taliesin, the great Bard of the Celts, sailed with Arthur as well. All along the way the Bard, who had first-hand knowledge of the Twilight Land, whispered into the King's ear tales from the Twilight Land. He told Arthur about treacherous enchantments, mystifying labyrinths and fierce warriors who could not die. He warned Arthur that his journey to the Twilight Land was fraught with peril and would only bring misery and despair.

"You do not want to enter the land of the Faery uninvited and plotting to steal their treasure," Taliesin warned.

Arthur shook off the Bard's grave counsel and steeled himself for battle with the Faery.

Some believed Arthur sailed to Ireland to combat the Faery. Others say it was Avalon. The old, very old, poem telling of Arthur's clash with the Faery and his theft of the Cauldron is vague about where the battle took place. But then again, twilight is a vague time of day. Let's journey with this story to the Isle of Avalon.

For many days and nights Arthur sailed until he

came to a place where thick spooky mist blinded his ships, clung to the cloaks of his men and clawed at their minds weaving uncertainty and dread. They sailed past seven islands shimmering like mirages, before they landed on the shores of Avalon.

Upon the isle, Arthur and his men fought six thousand silent soldiers before entering the Twilight of the Faery.

Little is told of Arthur's descent into the Land of the Faery. Some tales tell us Arthur finds the Cauldron of Annwn cradled in the arms of a Great Oak, The Tree of Life. The Oak's branches stretched high into the heavens and its roots penetrated deep into the underworld.

Tending to the Cauldron of Annwn were Nine Sisters. Morgan the Fey was one of the Nine Sisters, the keepers of the Ancient Earth Magic. Theirs was the most ancient magic known. It is the celebration of spring—crowning plants in damp soil and birds' song in the morning. It is the joy of summer— meadows of wildflowers and the fullness of green forest. It is the harvest of autumn—golden grains, trees ablaze and Orion's Belt shining in the night sky. It is the magic of winter—sparkling white stillness.

The Sisters, in rhythms old as time, sang ancient songs of Earth and swirled around the Cauldron that was dark as midnight and studded with glistening pearls. Their breath stirred the Cauldron of Annwn, bestowing it with magic carried in their hearts—gifts of poetic inspiration to nourish hunger and appease appetites.

Some say when Arthur spied the Cauldron greed rose in his heart and as he grasped the luminous vessel a spell was woven into his hand. He could not let go of the cauldron. Arthur bound to the cauldron by his own fear of scarcity made it easy for the Faery to catch their thief and throw him in prison, a labyrinth made of human bones.

For three days and three nights, all was lost. In the labyrinth's darkness, Arthur became muddled and dumb. Groans of dead soldiers condemned to the shadowy mists of Avalon tore his soul to pieces until on the third day he was rescued by two of his knights.

Arthur returned to Camelot. Only seven men disembarked onto the shores of Camelot. Each vowed never to speak of their time in the Twilight Land.

In mythologies all around the world, sacred trees, like the Oak, are doorways to both the riches and the despair of ancestors. These sacred trees offer two pathways: the path below and the path above. Roots of great old trees guide one on the path to the ancestors living below the Earth in the Underworld. Branches, reaching into the heaven, are climbed to seek the counsel of ancestors bathing in the sky's radiant light.

Follow the roots of a mighty Oak down into the Earth to find the troubled ancestors: the hungry, the angry, the beaten and the lost. These are the ancestors not spoken about. Their lives are the silent ones. They are silenced by the pain they bear. They cannot speak of the unspeakable acts they have witnessed, been subject to or perpetrated. Below, under the roots of benevolent Oak, the silence of intergenerational trauma is buried.

Unsettled ancestors living in the darkness of the underworld imprisoned by a labyrinth of bones can be found and healed by those living on the surface of the Earth. Those who live in the land that is neither above or below have the ability to travel across worlds, journey into Twilight Lands, and aid the ancestors who struggle in the darkness, muddled and confused, or who burn with malice, or hold on to all they have because letting go is unimaginable. There are two requirements if one chooses to follow a great tree's root down into the Underworld. One must be brave and have a good heart. Arthur, while he did not yet know it, had both.

Remember the Oak is ruled by Jupiter, the benevolent planet. The key to a journey into the Underworld is benevolence, knowledge of the goodness of life. It is the kindness in one's actions that Jupiter rewards.

Arthur, while young and feeling the need to prove himself, not yet knowing how to wear the robe of the king, was still a king. Jupiter rules kings. Kings are like guardians of doorways. A king's benevolence, or lack of, opens the door of war or peace, famine or contentment onto the lives of the people he serves.

Arthur is always described as a fair and just king. His benevolence was rewarded with the love of his people. Arthur's kindness, generosity of heart and bravery were qualities he was born with. He was also born with pride and self-doubt. His life experiences, like journeys into the Twilight Land tempered his more challenging qualities and strengthened the natural goodness of his heart.

Envision fearless Arthur disembarking from his ship

leading his loyal knights with fanfare and bravado only to come face to face with 6,000 voiceless soldiers: their missing limbs, bloody bandages and empty eyes standing in the mind-numbing mists of the Faery. I imagine Arthur's good heart crushed under the weight of the silence as he and his knights fought the 6,000 eerie shadows of men who had once been carpenters, farmers, black smiths, tavern owners, healers, poets, fathers, husbands and sons. Each man was a lost treasure buried in silence. The silence must have shaken Arthur, the leader of men. For how can a man lead shadows? A kingdom of silent men would be an impoverished kingdom indeed.

My thoughts turn to my own Grandmothers. They were silent women. My one Grandmother died when I was ten. I remember standing with her at the top of the wooden stairs in her small house while she opened the linen closet. From between carefully folded sheets, she took a miniature china tea pot wrapped in an embroidered hanky. She gave it to me with a warning not to tell anyone. There was a terrible silence in her house. Her house was always very clean. Like dust, no words gathered anywhere.

My other Grandmother went mad with loneliness. During the last five years of her life, she never said a word. Her lips would move, but no sounds came out.

Sometimes I feel like my Grandmothers' silence follows me through my life. Their silence is like the familiar face of a stranger I happen to glance on as I ride the subway, or pass under streetlights, or meet in my dreams as morning arrives. My Grandmothers' silence is in my blood. I appreciate American writer Joyce Carol Oats' statement, "We are linked by blood, and blood is memory without language." (Oates, 1990).

Blood is ruled by Jupiter, blood bringing the heart warmth and the rosy cheeks of good cheer. The warmth of the good life are gifts from Jupiter. Jupiter is not icy silence.

The Oak's medicine is blood medicine. It staunches bleeding and heals gangrene. Gangrene causes flesh to die and rot before the soul's death has arrived. The Oak's medicine binds edges of torn flesh and mends wounds. Washes of Oak bark slow creeping infection and speed the formation of scabs. A healing with Oak leaves very little scar tissue behind.

I cringe when people tell me that they need to deal with their emotions, or their illness, or their addiction, or whatever else it is they feel they need be rid of in their life. When people say they need to deal with sadness or anger, a terrible image arises in my mind of their emotions abandoned in a lonesome alley, amongst trash and bone-thin, hungry alley cats. When people tell me they need to deal with an illness images of them hacking off a limb or slicing off a piece of their flesh with a bloody serrated blade appear in my mind. And I want to tell them, but the difficult emotions, the painful illness, the compulsive addiction is part of you. If you pause for a moment and listen to its silence, you will find buried treasure.

History is like that. It silences the pain. Cuts it out. Leaves it behind. Abandons it to the haunted edges of dreams. We tell the story of the victors and edit out their brutality, cruelty, cold-heartedness. The lives of the hungry, the angry, the beaten and the lost are not told until some brave soul, with benevolence in his heart descends into the Underworld to stop the bleeding, bind the edges of torn souls and mend the wounds. It is the braveness in a good heart that returns warmth to blood and remembrance of the goodness of life.

My Grandmothers were more than their silence. My one Grandmother grew the most beautiful roses and baked the most wonderful cakes. She had an eye for beauty and the heart of an adventurer. My other Grandmother was soft with kindness. They both loved me so much. Something in their love always made me feel so special. Held in their loving gaze, I became a wonderful and unique child. Wrapped in my Grandmothers' love, only good things were possible. I am my Grandmothers' hope, and they are my hope.

My Great-Grandmother grew up near the Isle of Avalon. Surely, she knew the stories of Morgan the Fey and King Arthur, the Cauldron of Annwn and Nine Sisters' singing under the ancient Oak, the doorway to the ancestors.

I wonder if somewhere in my Grandmothers' silence whisps of the songs the Nine Sisters' sang still. It was the Sisters' swaying movements and the breath of their sacred songs that infused the Cauldron of Annwn with the magic of poetic inspiration. Inspired words of poets have carried human beings through the gravest hardships, the loneliest loss and rekindled Nature's beauty and abundance in the darkest of hearts. The Sister's magic woven deep, beyond where the eye can see and hands can reach right down to the roots of an ancient Oak, ignites wonder where there was once only hardship and pain.

Ancient Earth magic is full of wonder. It is the fierceness in the eyes of a woman pushing out new life. It is the amazement of seeing in a baby's twinkling eyes. It is the sweetness of an elder's smile and soulful eyes knowing all of what life brings. The Nine Sisters, with their songs and swirling dance around the ancient Oak, breathe the magic of life's abundance.

The essence of Earth magic is the elements: earth, water, fire and air. Ancient Earth teachings from all over the world are based in understanding the magic contained in the elements. For it is the continuous play of the elements, mingling this way, mixing that way, that creates the abundance of life in all its miraculous forms. Understanding the change that never changes is the doorway to a brave good heart.

The Oak Tree is a magnificent expression of the elements. The earth element offers the Oak sturdiness and finds itself in the hardness of the tree's wood. Oaks love water. Fifty percent of an ancient Oak's weight is water. They store water during drought, quenching the thirst of the plants that grow around its roots. When there is an abundance of rain, they release water back into the air to be carried on the wind and offered to dry places. It is their love of water that brings the Oak fire. There is a turbulent love affair between fire and water. Oak is left burnt and hollowed out by lightening fire. It is these empty places in the heart of the Oak that shelter many small animals and birds. Finally, there is air, playing in the Oaks green leaves, whispering of times past and times to come.

In a circle the Nine Sisters spin, round and round the ancient Oak chanting, intoning the wealth of earth, the many faces of water, fire's passion, hot and cold, and air's journey through time. The Nine Sisters carried the magic of Earth's songs. They knew the songs that heal and the songs that wound. The Sisters' wisdom songs told the beginnings in endings and the endings in beginnings. The Nine Sister's songs sow the seeds of seasons past into the seeds of future seasons. Their songs fill the Cauldron of Annwn with Plenty.

In Earth Magic, the elements make all possible. The elements are the myriad dances of Nature. No one is separate from them. Every form spins in and out of being as water clings to earth and fire ignites desire while air sends all along their way. All is created by Nature and all will return to Nature. The Nine Sisters sing this truth. They sing that every life is a flower, a river, the wind. Their dance, circling round and round the ancient tree, was a dance of deathlessness, only changing form and changing form and changing form. The Nine Sisters sang songs of flowers becoming goddesses, trees forming fingers and words creating form.

This is the teaching of Jupiter. Earth Magic is the abundance of Jupiter.

Jupiter brings benevolence because there is only benevolence. Beginnings are endings. Death is birth. Poverty can be reversed with a handful of seeds or a heart full of kind words. Mighty Oaks grow from tiny acorns. When deeply rooted and reaching high in the sky, the Oak mends wounds and holds space for the troubled and the contented, the grief stricken and the joyous, the bitter and the kind. Journeys of a brave good heart to the Underworld bring treasure. Listen to the wind and sing the songs of Grandmothers. Open the door to magic.

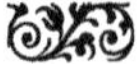

JUPITER, BEAUTY, AND BORAGE

Jupiter is the "Great Benefactor" of the solar system. Jupiter's vibration is equated with the good life, opportunities and expansion. Jupiter is not about living in a small way. Jupiter pushes aside the same old ways of doing things and welcomes the new. Jupiter is just, fair and kind. Jupiter is thoughtful, noble and generous. When Jupiter arrives, change comes for the better.

Who does not love good things, change for the better, more beauty and noble sentiments? No one I know. The problem is, we do not all agree on what is good, noble and beautiful. The planet of good fortune also carries the warning, "Be careful what you wish for."

Wishes are for the future. When we think about meeting 'the one', or the next step up in a career, or believe in the new house where we'll be happy, Jupiter is at play. Jupiter arrives with the future.

The future creeps into every moment with its hope and uncertainty. The beautiful, problematic future is fuelled by today's plots and plans, wishes and fears, rewards and losses. The future remains both wished for and feared. The future describes a time when everything is possible, and nothing is known.

This was Helen of Troy's problem. She longed for a future where she could be free to choose whom she loved, go where she wanted to go and be more than a pretty face. Like a bird in a gilded cage, Helen was entrapped by the good things in life: status, power and wealth.

As the Queen of Sparta, Helen's life was safe and the palace routines monotonous. Her words and sentiments were scripted by the duty of her position. Her marriage was predictable. Every day was organized and arranged around court rituals and ceremonies. To make matters worse, Helen was The Most Beautiful Woman in the World. Her beauty encased her heart in a luminous shell. It was nearly impossible to see beyond the glamour her beauty cast, nearly impossible to peer into her soul. Helen was lonely, frustrated and wanting more.

Beauty is a blessing we are told. We expect people with beautiful faces to be healthier, more intelligent, more trustworthy and to have more friends than those who are average looking. Humans have powerful physiological responses to beauty. Hearts race. Words are lost. Hormones surge. We blush and feel faint. It is easy to become lost in beauty and miss the person behind the beautiful face.

There is one more challenge beauty brings. Beauty is a commodity.

Helen yearned for recklessness, adventure and

passion. Helen needed to wake up in a world where everything was new and unpredictable. She craved spontaneous laughter and meaningful, heartfelt confessions. She needed the soft strokes of a lover's fingertips to send shivers sparking across her skin. Helen of Sparta longed for life beyond the walls of her palace. When a beautiful man astute enough to understand her longings offered her a chance to fulfill her desires, Helen's future had arrived.

To understand Helen's future, we must turn to her past. For the future is contained in the past and the past is contained in the future. Jupiter vibrates with this truth, a truth some call karma. Jupiter is the planet of justice—what is sown is what is harvested.

To appreciate Helen's desire and the pull of her beauty we must begin with her father, Zeus, whom the Romans later called Jupiter. For the Romans and the Greeks, there was no higher god than Zeus. He was the supreme leader of all the gods in the Greek pantheon. When supplicating Zeus, Greeks called him Father.

Zeus first appeared in sacred stories from India that told tales about the exploits of elemental gods: Earth, Sky, Fire, Water and Wind. In these sacred texts called the Rigveda, Zeus was named Dyaus. Dyaus was a Sky God. But he was not just the Sky, boundless and vast. Dyaus was the constant light that radiated throughout sky, no matter its colour or mood.

To get a feel for this, imagine a bright blue summer sky. You are lying on the grass. The air is warm on your skin and the earth below is cool on your back. Open your eyes and gaze into vast, empty sky. Let its brightness penetrate your eyes and pour into your body. Let the sky's light infuse every cell of your being and fill your mind. For a moment, disappear into the sky.

When you return you feel peaceful, expansive and full of love. There is a brightness in you. The brightness is now forever part of you. You have just been blessed by Jupiter. The ancients would say, "You have been impregnated by Zeus."

When personified as a man, Zeus is lascivious, or even worse, a rapist. He has no control over his all-encompassing lust. Zeus pursues women to the ends of the Earth, ravishes them and leaves behind his seed swelling in their wombs.

When personified as a god, Zeus is a numinous procreative power. He is an initiating force. Throwing thunderbolts, Zeus impregnates the great Mother Earth with the fire of creativity. His rain awakens Earth's many seeds.

Zeus' extravagant fertility manifests in many forms. To plant his seed, his potency takes on flesh as a bull, eagle, vulture, ant, bear, serpent, or star. In the stories contained in Greek Mythology he fathered between 130 to 150 children with goddesses, nymphs, and mortal women. His procreative drive expresses the many passions of sex: love and tenderness, need and lust, violence and rage, power and commerce, humiliation and punishment. Zeus' stories are not really about sex between a god and women. They tell the story of the undying passionate creative force that pervades this planet.

Zeus is the creative power that sired Helen. With

the prolific, adventurous Zeus as her father, how would it be possible for Helen to play it safe, follow the script and be content in a gilded cage?

The identity of Helen's mother depends on whether you are reading the Iliad or its precursor the Cypria. The Iliad was recorded by a Greek storyteller Homer. It tells the stories of men who became heroes during the Trojan war.

The spark that ignited the Trojan war was Helen. When Helen fell for a handsome prince from a rival royal family, the Trojans, and left behind her role as the Spartan Queen, wife, and mother to run off with him, war was declared. The Cypria, attributed to the poet named Stasinus, is about the years leading up to the war.

It is important to remember that the Trojan War happened five hundred years before either Homer or Stasnius were born. The stories the poets eventually recorded had been passed down for five centuries in an oral tradition. This led to many different versions of the same story. The details told and the details left out depended on what was to be gained and what was to be lost.

Jupiter's expansiveness holds many different points of view.

Throughout the stories of the Trojan War, there is no singular Helen. Some poets are sympathetic towards her, others tell her story with contempt, while others portray her as a helpless victim of circumstances.

Depending on which poet is telling her story, Helen has different mothers. In one version her mother is the

Queen of Sparta, Leda. Leda was seduced by Zeus when he took the form of a majestic swan. Later she laid the egg from which Helen hatched.

My preferred mother for Helen is the Goddess Nemesis, the Goddess of Retribution. She is the dark-faced Goddess, daughter of Justice. It is Nemesis who determines the punishment of those who violate the natural order of nature. She is particularly merciless to those who shame and humiliate others to enhance their sense of superiority. Nemesis' acts of retribution are scattered throughout Helen's story.

Zeus desired Nemesis. Zeus was Nemesis' father and his advances brought shame to her heart, so she fled from him. She raced across the land and plunged into the sea shifting her shape into many different animals desperate to confuse her hunter. Zeus relentlessly stalked her. When he spied her as a goose enjoying the cool waters of a river under a willow tree, he became a magnificent swan and descended. Nemesis was powerless against his strength.

Following the rape, Nemesis laid an egg. Hermes, also known as Mercury, took the egg and dropped it into Leda's lap. Leda cared for the egg until it hatched and out sprang Helen. Leda and her husband, the King of Sparta, Tyndareus, adopted her. It was Tyndareus who coined the phrase, the Most Beautiful Woman on Earth, to describe Helen. He used it to promote a contest for her hand in marriage. Her adopted father knew the desire of men. What man would not want to possess the Most Beautiful Woman in the World? It was a great marketing ploy.

But we are ahead of ourselves. Let's return to Helen the girl. She is a child conceived during rape, living in a foster home. Imagine the secrets whispered about her behind closed doors. From whom does she get her beauty? Is she worth all the trouble it took to raise her to be a Queen? Would her uncertain genes make an appearance and spoil all the planning and expense? Should we tell her who she really is?

Consider the uncertainty those whispers planted in Helen's heart. The unspoken words, the sense that there was something amiss with her, not normal, hidden, would have left behind a tender bruise, a soft ache when touched in Helen's heart. She would have been driven to prove herself as a good and dutiful daughter. She had to show the court she was worthy of all her foster parents had bestowed upon her.

To complicate matters, Helen, as we already know, was an exceptional beauty. Her beauty even as an adolescent stirred desire in the loins of men. There is a side story few poets tell in detail about something that happened before Helen's marriage and her affair. As an adolescent she was abducted by a man named Theseus. Most poets write that Theseus was a young man when he stole Helen from her family.

Bettany Hughes, historian and expert on all things Helen, tells another story. In Bettany's version of events, Helen was raped on a riverbank by Theseus who at the time was a 70-year-old man. There are even hints that during the rape a child was conceived, a little girl named Iphigenia, who was given to Helen's older sister to raise. (Hughes. 2015).

After the rape Helen is a girl who no longer feels she has autonomy over her body. That is what rape does to girls. It steals a girl's body. It robs girls of the intrinsic truth their bodies contain. There is a loss of connection with the body's wisdom. After rape, being embodied becomes dangerous. It is better not to feel the pain and confusion, rage and grief, violation and betrayal. It is easier to surrender to feelings of numbness. So much is forgotten following rape. Rape turns a girl into a ghost of her former self.

Most stories about Helen offer the listener a mere word or two about this time in her life. I have read none that consider the effects Theseus actions would have had on Helen and her choices later in life. Girls who are raped often try to be really good until they become tired of feeling numb and throw all caution to the wind.

Tyndareus decided to marry Helen off as quickly as possible after the rape, before whispers of Theseus' crime turned Helen into spoiled goods. Her beauty was still a great commodity and he wanted it sold at a high price.

When Tyndareus announced the competition for Helen's hand, men gathered from all over Mycenaea to offer lavish gifts and demonstrate their great strength. Having Helen as a wife promised increased wealth and power, for she came from a great family. And there was also the added bonus of Helen's beauty. What man would not want something all other men desired—The Most Beautiful Woman in the World.

Tyndareus feared fighting might break out between the many men who had gathered to win Helen as their trophy. He was afraid there might be sore losers who would rise up against the man he chose for Helen and war would break out. To avoid this, Tyndareus asked each man to take an oath to defend the man he chose to marry Helen against any challenger.

After the oath was taken by each man, Menelaus, the younger brother of the war-loving and powerful King Agamemnon was given to Helen and a great political marriage was made.

Menelaus was much older than Helen. He was a kind man, thoughtful and considerate. He was also dull. Shortly after their marriage, Helen gave birth to a girl she named Hermione.

And time passed for Helen. More time passed for Helen. No more children were born. Helen watched her husband age and her youth begin to slip away. She wandered the palace dreaming of a life beyond its cold stone walls. At night she imagined a lover of her own choosing, not a tired man who came to her out of duty by night and by day paraded her about as a trophy for all the world to see. She wanted a handsome, vital, daring man, who would throw duty aside for reckless adventure. She wanted to feel alive. She needed to feel.

One day, when Helen was about 24 years old a Trojan prince arrived at the palace gates. The prince's name was Paris. The story goes Aphrodite, the Goddess of Love, had promised Paris Helen, for he too desired The Most Beautiful Woman in the World.

Paris, under the guise of a diplomatic mission offered Menelaus and Helen gifts finer that any found within their palace walls. His eyes flirted with Helen.

Helen was smitten. Sparks flew, love was made and Helen woke with possibilities she had dared not dream of before. Her future had finally arrived. She fled the known for the unknown.

Breathless, having finally tasted sexual pleasure, the thrill of travel, the recklessness of adventure, Helen arrived in Troy, the greatest, richest, multi-cultural city of the ancient world.

Ah! Jupiter promises big and forgets the details. Someone should have told Helen about the active sex trade that ran through Troy and the harem of women, the wives, concubines and sex slaves (the spoils of war) that shared Paris' bed. Someone should have told Helen that great sex doesn't guarantee a meaningful relationship.

After the orgasm, you still have to sit across from each other at the breakfast table and find something to talk about. It wasn't long before Helen realized Paris was a peacock and she was once more a trophy. But that was the least of Helen's worries.

War followed her to Troy. Remember the oath to defend the man who was given Helen. The Mycenean warriors, bored with peace and fearing their lives would end before songs could be written about their battlefield heroics, found in Helen's folly a reason to go to war. They loaded up their chariots and warhorses on ships and sailed across the Aegean Sea to the shores of Troy beating their chests and drums. Finally, they were off to war. They too had dreamed of adventure.

The army that followed Helen did not endear her to the Trojans. Paris' mother spits at her:

My son Paris was a heart-stopping boy,
And you, adulterous witch, wanted him.
And he was rich. Your heart flew at that.
Your husband here, King Menelaus, had a nice, modest castle;
You'd heard about our palaces – luxurious, lofty –
So-long Menelaus, Paris – come on in! (Euripides. 412 BC).

HELEN'S DREAMS OF ADVENTURE AND A GREAT LOVE affair became soaked in the blood from the battles raging outside the gates of Troy and smothered by the shame and blame heaped upon her by Trojans and Greeks alike. Living in Troy, Helen became known as the greatest whore in all the world. In Troy, Helen was utterly alone. She cried, "Wherefore I wail alike for thee and for my hapless self with grief at heart; for no longer have I anyone beside in broad Troy that is gentle to me or kind; but all men shudder at me."

Nine years later, Paris died on the battlefield. The Council of Trojan Elders voted to give Helen back to the Greeks and be done with her and the war she had brought to their shores. Paris' brother, Diephobos, felt entitled to the time-honoured tradition of taking a brother's widow for a wife. Helen became another man's trophy and was bound to a brute of a man, one who used her as a weapon against the Greeks.

When the Greeks offered the Trojans a gift of a

massive wooden horse, Diephobos senses deception. I can imagine him gripping Helen by the hair as they circle around the wooden horse, him pushing her, demanding she call out to the men he suspects are inside. He insists Helen mimic the voices of their wives longing for their return. When no sounds comes from the belly of the wooden horse, Diephobos is satisfied it is not filled with Greeks.

Some stories claim Helen knew there were Greek warriors hiding in the belly of the horse. Some say she was as invested as Diephobos in ferreting out the true purpose of the horse. I don't believe this latter is true.

At this point in the story, Helen's dreams of romance and adventure are shattered. She must have longed for a place where she could find peace with herself. For ten long years, Helen had lived among people who cursed her as their enemy. She had watched the slaughter of men from Troy's walls. She had been tossed aside by her handsome prince and forced to share the bed with a man she hated.

During that ten years, Helen had had time to consider her life with Menelaus, the price of her recklessness and the wisdom gained from mistakes. She must have yearned once more for a new future, a future that celebrated peace. When the Greeks arrived inside the gates of Troy, Helen's future arrived once more.

The Trojans brought the wooden horse into their city accepting it as a peace offering. They believed the gift of the big, beautiful horse was a gesture of surrender from the Greeks. They uncorked the wine and partied. They drank and danced in victory until the early hours of morning. When the city was quiet and the Trojans were sleeping off their drunken celebration, the Greeks crept from the belly of the horse and slaughtered the Trojans while setting fire to their magnificent city.

Menelaus, seeking honour after being the cuckold, burst into Diephobos bedchamber and chopped him up into pieces. First, he sliced off Diephobos' ears, then his nose. Next, he hacked off Diephobos' arms and finally his legs. Drenched in bloody murder and thirsty for more, Menelaus raged through the burning city bawling Helen's name, demanding that he be the one to kill her.

He found Helen trapped in an ally's dead end, huddled against a stone wall, surrounded by Greeks and Trojans alike. They spat on her, calling her a whore. They gathered rocks to stone her. Menelaus demanded again his right to kill her. The crowd, overwhelmed by the blood-soaked mad man wielding his sword stepped back. As Menelaus raised his sword to slice Helen in two, she dropped the shoulder of her gown revealing a breast. Menelaus crumbled to the ground. Electra, Menelaus' niece, who was in the crowd cried, "Can it be that her beauty has blunted their swords?"

The day after, Helen and Menelaus boarded a small sailboat and took to the seas. The hurt each carried was thicker than all the clotted blood that had been shed during the ten year war. Having no direction home, they sailed aimlessly over the Aegean Sea. After thirsty, hot days at sea, they landed on the shores of Egypt. The Egyptian Queen took them in.

Helen confided in the Queen, "My life and fortunes

are a monstrosity... partly because of my beauty. I wish I had been wiped clean like a painting and made plain instead of beautiful." (Euripides, 412 BC).

Menelaus spent his days drowning his sorrows in beer, weeping over the bloodshed and raging over Helen's betrayal. They could not meet each other's eyes.

The Queen of Egypt, a woman of experience and wisdom saw in Helen a woman with many sorrows. She offered to help Helen let go of her pain and embrace a new life. The Queen gave Helen a cup of Nepenthe, the medicine of forgetting.

Some modern scholars say Nepenthe was opium. Other believe it was a blend of Henbane and opium. I think Pliny the Elder and Dioscorides, a Greek herbalist from around the same time as Christ, were correct when they wrote Nepenthe is an infusion of Borage.

Upon Helen and Menelaus' arrival on her doorstep, the Queen may have offered them a draught of opium to sleep. Sleep is a balm for those trembling with fear, shaking with rage and tormented by hurt. Opium numbs pain for a night or day but when the plant's effects wear off, there is only a stupor in the mind while the horrors of the past remain. Opium is not a solution when one cannot look another in the eye. It is a momentary reprieve from pain.

Henbane brings visions of wonder and horror. Like most other psychoactive plants, it purges the mind of its trouble. But it can also easily overwhelm the mind's connection to the body leading to madness. I can't see Henbane being helpful to a man and woman trying to find their way back to each other's heart. I can't see a blend of the forgetfulness of opium and the visions of Henbane bestowing the heart with the courage needed to forgive after so much hurt and so many losses.

Borage, a plant ruled by Jupiter, bestows courage.

When Borage's star-shaped flowers open at dawn, they are pink and gaze up at the sky. As the sun rises, the flowers turn sky blue and seem to be infused with a shimmering light of the sky. It's like the flowers are kissed by the boundless light that permeates the sky no matter its mood.

As the flowers turn to sky blue, they become heavier and begin to droop. Herbalists teach that the drooping blue flowers are a sign of medicine that uplifts heavy hearts and eases burdens. Borage's sky-blue flower helps the heart recall the boundless creative vibrancy of life, Jupiter's blessing.

A heavy heart is weighted with depression. A heavy heart is void of Jupiter's expansive optimism. A heavy heart does not carry the courage to grasp life's ever-changing opportunities. A heavy heart does not have the clarity of mind to recognize the law of karma at work.

Borage with its dropping sky-blue flowers fortifies the heart with courage and brings clarity to the mind after the reality of naive wishes, rash actions and foolish choices bring blame and shame, regrets and loss, hurt and confusion. Borage carries the medicine to remember the fragility of the human heart and the courage to forgive.

Forgiveness is not about forgetting the past. The

future is planted in the past. To forget is to risk making the same mistakes over and over again. Forgiveness is about opening to a life more expansive than trauma and pain. Forgiveness allows all of life, the good and the bad, to be bathed in the beauty contained within every human heart.

Borages' flowers have been used for a very long time in this way. Nepenthe, an infusion of these sky-blue flowers, is a potion that soothes terrible hurts and reconnects the heart with life's dynamic dance of creativity.

Helen and Menelaus drank their cups of Borage tea and found the courage to look each other in the eye. They opened to the pain, the regret and the love in each other. The cup of star-shaped flowers guided Helen and Menelaus back to the purity of their hearts where they found forgiveness. Forgiveness is the expansive expression of Jupiter, the magnanimous planet.

Helen's future arrived once more as she returned to Greece with Menelaus and they settled down for a quiet life. Over time, the warriors Menelaus had fought side by side with came to visit. Helen saw the hollow look in their eyes and felt the coldness in their hearts left behind by the war's brutality. She knew the despair of not being able to turn back time and choose another path.

Helen, understanding the old warriors' pain, brewed them a tea infused with Borage flowers. As she handed them the medicine, she shone the warmth of her beauty onto them and melted the icy hatred in their hearts. Helen, after all the longings, disappointments, shame and sorrow understood the blessings of her beauty. Borage renewed the courage in the old warriors' hearts while Helen's beauty inspired them to love again.

The rest of Helen and Menelaus' lives were not particularly interesting. There were no more affairs or wars. Jupiter, however, did not abandon them but bestowed upon them the greatest blessing of all, the good fortune to care for the beauty in another's heart.

SATURN, OLD WOMEN, AND BELLADONNA

When someone suggests I rest in the present moment, I scratch my head and wonder, "Where's that at?"

Time expands and contracts, seems boundless, endless, forever or becomes as tight as a pair of shoes that are one size too small. And just when it seems there's enough time to stop for gas on the way to work, call your mother or sit down and enjoy a cup of tea, it disappears. How can you rest in a moment that is constantly disappearing, again and again and again? That is no place to rest.

Saturn, the keeper of time out there, spinning on the rim of the inner solar system, marks the edge where time becomes numbers so vast they are meaningless. And here is Saturn's paradox. We are all living with limited time. Our time will come. But what is on the other side of that limit we do not know. Saturn teaches whatever the limit, there is always another side.

Time has not always been measured by hours,

minutes, moments. It was during the industrial revolution that lives began to be measured in minutes and hours to fit the rhythms of factories' input and output.

Time became linear when people left their small villages that had existed since before time was remembered and poured into cities seeking work. Before the factories and the cities, time was measured by the swelling of a sheep's belly, acorns falling, and Orion's Belt rising in the sky. Time was eternal change that never changes, like the cycle of the moon - dark moon, waxing moon, full moon, waning moon, dark moon, and on and on, endlessly.

There was a time when we waited for the cows to home before having dinner. Days began at sunrise and nights arrived with sunset. The sharp honk of geese in the sky brought beginnings and endings. Hawthorn blooms welcomed in long days sweet with Sun's warmth. Squash ripening on their tangled vines announced the arrival of dark nights and long stories. Each moment was once marked and named by a whiff of Valerian's sticky sweet smell, the rise of cumulus clouds or the first snow flake. Nature's cycles announced the change of time with a language of bird calls, scents on the winds and changes of light.

Nature's language of change is understood by those who pause, take in the landscape and watch season after season arrive with predictability. Yet, like any language, Nature's language carries nuance, veiled meanings, and uncertainty, "Is that what this really meant?"

Nature's hidden language is felt in the presence of a landscape. Nature's language is filled with vast silences punctuated by moments between the loon's longing call rising from dawn's mist-covered lakes or the woodpecker's staccato on the old Oak out back. Nature's meaning is found in the unspoken presence of place.

It is in the silence between dried leaves scattered by the autumn breeze and the trickle of spring's running waters that I find spaces to rest. Nature's sounds define the limits of the known; its silences announce the limits of the unknown. It is in the space between the known and unknown that I let go and just breathe. This is Saturn's blessing.

The Celts told stories about an Old Woman who breathed the sweet air of the islands that have been surrounded by the North Sea since the oceans were forests and the mountains were valleys. She knew the veiled language of Nature. She, like Saturn, carried the blessing of the space between the known and the unknown.

Not long ago, a priest knocked on the Old Woman's door to ask her age. The Old, very old Woman, shrugged her shoulders and yawned. "What does it matter?" she asked, her voice a sigh as soft as water's ebb and flow.

The priest, being a man who believed in answers and only understood linear time, was puzzled by her response. "Of course, it matters," he reassured the Old Woman, reassuring himself.

"If you need to know, go into my attic and count the bones," and she pointed with her long, crooked finger, nails rimmed with the dirt of time, to a ladder propped up next to the door. "You'll find a bone for every year I have walked this land."

So, the priest climbed the ladder and began to count bones. One bone, two bones, three bones. Soon he had counted a hundred bones.

"A hundred years old is a mighty fine age," he mumbled to himself as he turned to go down the ladder. Just as he was about to place his foot on the ladder's first rung, hundreds of bones rattled and tumbled into the attic. The priest resumed his counting.

The priest counted and counted, all day and all night. Just when he thought the attic was empty, another clamour sounded, as bones, long and white, covered the attic floor. Obsessed with getting to the bottom of this strange attic full of strange bones and the strange old woman sitting below by the fire, the priest counted for weeks that became months. One day he was found wandering, mad, across the mountain where the Old Woman lived, counting.

The Old Woman is very old. Some say she has existed since the long eternity of the world. Others say this is not true. First there was Salmon, then there was Otter, followed by Eagle and finally the Old Woman.

If you ask her about a long time ago, and she does not recall, she will send you first to speak to Eagle, then to Otter and finally Salmon who was here at the beginning of it all. The Old Woman's name is the Cailleach Beira, most often called the Cailleach or just the Hag.

The Cailleach is fearsome to look upon. She has only one eye, but the sight of it is keen and sharp as ice and as swift as the mackerel in the ocean. Her face is etched with lines like a craggy mountain top. Her complexion is dull, dusk blue.

Her teeth are red as rust. Her locks fall heavily on her shoulders. They curl and swirl like the eddies in a whirlpool and are as white as aspen covered in hoar-frost. On her head there is a cap like old women used to wear long ago. Some say under her cap deer antlers sprout.

Her clothing is home spun, dyed the brown colours of heather on an early spring day. She is never seen without her great fringed shawl, drawn closely round her shoulders.

She wears seashells for earrings. If you look closely you will see bits and pieces of seaweed, long dried, in her hair. Her eye shines with the light of the Sun and the Moon.

When you pause next to a solitary standing stone on a cliff to watch ocean's rise and fall, or kneel at the edge of a deep spring with a prayer in your heart, it is the Cailleach put them there. The stones and spring are her words speaking the presence of place. Since before memory she has traveled the land, carrying stones in her apron, dropping one here and one there. Her stones have shaped mountains and valleys, lakes and rivers, islands and cairns for the dead.

All over the land, there are places she made that bear her name. On the Isle of Sky there is *Beinn na Caillich* ('Mountain of the Cailleach') and in Ireland there is the *Ceann Caillíin* ('Hag's Head'). The whirlpool where she does her washing, near the Isle of Bute, Scotland is simply called the Cailleach. Her chair, a large flat stone with armrests sits on a hill called Slieve na Calliagh. Her bed is an ancient tomb found in a farmer's field near County Cork, Ireland. Her footprints mark rocky paths through mountain ranges and can be seen where once she slid down cliffs to the seaside.

You can hardly travel anywhere over the great hills and valleys of Scotland and Ireland without encountering the Cailleach who made a lake there and carved a river here. You may even hear her named on the wind as snowflakes begin to fall—CAILLAECH. It is the Cailleach who, using a thread of tangled knots, summons winds wild with winter and winds warm with spring.

The Cailleach cares for all animals, but has a particular fondness for deer, owls and eagles. Some have seen her take Eagle's shape and soar. Others say she was once a Deer who became a woman to marry a man. She brought her husband great wealth. After his betrayal, she returned to the skin of Deer, leapt over fences and disappeared up the mountainside taking her wealth with her.

Even though she cherishes her deer, the Cailleach will help a hunter. She understands all have hunger. She will show the hunter the weakest deer and make the kill easy. But if the hunter becomes greedy, her wrath will arrive with a sudden storm of ice and hail and knee-deep snow. The hunter's body will be found in the spring, cowering, frozen solid.

Some say it was the Cailleach who gave humans their upright stance. The marrow in the spine bones is named for her: smior-cailleach. The Cailleach catches the babe as she emerges from the womb. It is the Cailleach's touch that shapes the spine and makes the babe helpless, only walking after a year or so of life and many bumps and falls.

She pays a visit to each boy and girl as they transform into man and woman. The Cailleach leaves behind wavy translucent scars on young hips and thighs where her touch urged them to grow. Her fingers leave the same marks on the bellies of pregnant woman.

The Cailleach is everywhere, in everything.

Every hundred years, the Cailleach must return to the sea to be renewed. This is the secret of her old, very old, age. Legend tells she must enter the water at dawn before the first dog barks or else she dies. Even the Cailleach has limits within her timelessness.

This year was a year that the Cailleach needed to return to the sea. As she descended her mountain at dawn, for she left early to be sure to make it to sea before the dog barked, she heard a great roar, a crack like something breaking and a terrible grinding sound.

The noise frightened her, and she rushed down the mountainside in her crooked old woman way to see what was the matter. Soon she came upon the ugly destruction of a clearcut forest. Hidden in the crevice of a nearby cliff, she watched trucks haul the wealth of trees down a spiral carved into the mountainside. She could not believe her eyes and wanted to stop, but she had to make her way to the sea before it was too late.

So, the Cailleach walked on and soon a strange thunder rumbled across the mountain, the air became thick with dust and under her feet the earth shook. The Cailleach almost fell from the shock of it all. Again, she hurried down the mountainside in her crooked old woman way to see what was the matter. It was not long before she saw that the side of the mountain had been cut away, and again trucks hauling away the mountain's wealth rumbled down a new spiralling path carved into the mountain side.

Again, the Cailleach wanted to stop. But she had to make her way to the sea before it was too late.

The Cailleach, confused, the weight of the destruction on her heart, walked on and on and came upon a hard, hot path running through a wide valley. Her feet burned as she walked along this strange new path. She looked to either side of the long, hard hot path and where once wild flowers danced, bees buzzed and her beloved deer grazed, there was now a plant with a yellow flower. For miles and miles, the same yellow flower, Cannola, bloomed. The land had become yellow. The scent of the flower made her head feel heavy and her muscles ache. Cailleach slowed for she could not breathe the air with gentleness but had to force it into her lungs. Step by step she passed through this strange yellow valley devoid of wildflowers, bees and deer.

Around a curve she walked and saw something lying on the path. She bent to take a closer look. It was a little fox. Its back was broken and one leg flattened. She knelt and tenderly touched the little fox, wishing to ease its pain. Tears crept from her eyes and where they fell a little pile of rocks formed to mark the tiny creature's passing.

It was getting late and the Cailleach still had a way to go. All night long she walked through a vast city with swirling lights, choking fumes and cracked, grey paths where people slept in rags while others scurried by with empty eyes.

When Venus appeared on the horizon announcing the imminence of dawn's arrival, the Cailleach smelled the sea. She paused on the cliff overlooking the beach where she had entered the water every hundred years and saw the sand was no longer golden brown. It was coloured with bits of red and green, purple and orange. As far as her eye could see, the beach was littered with lengths of yellow rope and blue toothbrushes and black rubber soles of shoes scattered among empty white tampon tubes. Everywhere clear water bottles were filled with sand. A headless Barbie doll and bright red pail lay in a tangled clump of dried seaweed. At her feet a tiny crab scampered by wearing a pink bottle cap as her home. The Cailleach paused bewildered. And a dog barked.

As old stories call Cailleach the Old Woman, astrologers call Saturn the Old Man, the Elder amongst the planets. Astrologers tell us that if a life has been lived honestly Saturn brings sobering wisdom gained from making mistakes. Saturn is the Old Man who understands the limits of ambition and greed. Saturn is the Old Man who knows his life is sure to end in death. Saturn is the Old Man who wonders what is on the other side.

For 3,000 years astronomers believed Saturn was the edge of the known human universe. Saturn is the last of the inner planets -those visible to the naked eye. For a very long time, humans have gazed upon Saturn, a distant light veiled by time and space, coming and going from the nighttime sky. Saturn, with its cool distance, was the edge of the known world. It was the rim on the container for human awareness. Since humans first glimpsed Saturn they have been telling stories about what lies beyond its limits. Saturn is a boundary that fills the imagination with the unfamiliar. The Cailleach, like Saturn, is the edge between the known and the unknown.

While Cailleach marks the landscape with her familiar mountains, rivers, lakes and standing stones, she herself is completely unfamiliar. She is not a Goddess. She is too untamed and multifaceted to be a Goddess. Some say she is Mother Nature. But Salmon swam, Otter played and Eagle took flight before she arrived. Some believe she is an ancient Earth Spirit. The oldest translation of her name is the Veiled One. The Cailleach exists behind a veil. She is unseen. To be unseen is be unknown, unfamiliar and perhaps inviting chaos.

Veils blur distinctions. They cast doubt on familiarity. We can't really believe our eyes when looking through a veil. Veils define the limits of knowing. Cailleach, like Saturn, marks the boundary between the known and the unknown, the familiar and the unfamiliar, the predictable and the chaos, meaning and meaninglessness. Saturn and Cailleach are containers for the known beyond which lies the unknown.

Stories are containers. Stories, like healers, hold space for the grief and joy of life. Stories provide beginnings and endings and, in the middle, allow in just enough chaos to shift perspective, plant the seed for a new relationship and perhaps breathe a little easier.

My writing mentor Charlene Jones says, "You need to make your reader feel safe. Give them a good beginning, a decent ending and in between carry them from idea to idea. Structure will keep your reader safe." This is what Saturn does. It provides structure, a container. Containers have limits. Every story has its limit. Every limit is surrounded by the limitless. This is the teaching of both Saturn and the stories of the Cailleach with her stones and footprints left behind on mountain passes, creating a container within the vast wilderness.

The story of my life is a restless one. Life has taken me here and there. Sometimes I will stop for a while, but eventually I am on the move again. Restless, I have always been envious of people whose lives are rimmed with landmarks, like my elderly neighbour whose life is circled by landmarks I cannot see. He tells me the path to the Hawthorns runs past the old Mackenzie house. All that is left of the Mackenzie house are a few foundation stones in a patch of Nettles and my neighbour's memories of times past. He tells me it was Mackenzie's wife that planted the trees. He can no longer recall her name.

I have never known a landscape with the intimacy of time. Landmarks have not defined the edges of my known restless story.

Before the landscape was marked by foundation stones of houses that no longer stand, it was Cailleach who defined the landscape, making it known. With her apron full of stones, her winds and storms, Cailleach left her name in untamed places building containers in the unknown with stones and rivers. She left behinds hills and lakes creating a language that tells the story of the land, offering a familiar place to rest in the wilderness.

Sitting by a warm hearth, the only light on a cold dark night, it must have been comforting to know that out in the wild somewhere a woman old as the hills walked, tending herds of deer. When blustery winds rattled windows and drafts seeped in under the door, telling stories of the Cailleach summoning storms with her knotted string would have been soothing. Every story has an ending, as does every storm. Seeing where her long fingers scored the rocks on a high mountain pass must have been reassuring that there was a place named in the wilderness. Her placement of stones on the cliff must have brought certainty, a kind of safety to a land where winter takes life and spring arrives with hunger. Her stones gave language to the veiled story of the land. The Cailleach with her weird feral timelessness offered landmarks in the uncertainty of life.

When the noblemen came to the place where the Cailleach's stones tell tales passed down from fathers and mothers, they told my ancestors to leave. The noblemen had done the calculations and discovered sheep were more profitable than people. My ancestors replied, "But, my Lords, we belong here. This is the place where the bones of our ancestors lie."

The noblemen unrolled a piece of paper and showed the people their deeds. "This is not about bones and belonging," the noblemen said. "We own the land."

When the people refused to leave the place where

the Cailleach had carefully placed her circles of stones, the noblemen let loose their dogs. The people ran, dogs at their heels, the smoke of their burning homes filling their lungs. I have been restless ever since, seeking the place where my ancestors' bones lie and I know the old stories contained in stones and rivers, the language of the curious scratches on the side of a hill and songs of the wind. For a long time, I have been seeking the place that defines my known world. I do not need a present moment to rest in, I need a place that knows my bones.

Saturn rules bones: the ulna's hard round rise as it joins the wrist, the long steady descent of the shin bone, the valley of the clavicles at the base of the throat. It is the protuberance of bones that defines the landscape of the skin. Bones are the last part of us to decay. When unearthed bones tell the story of our lives long after our names have disappeared.

Old women feel their bones more keenly than the young do. Their bones ache. Their bones creak and grind. The bumps and curves of their bones are easily traced under thin skin. Perhaps it is because of the groaning in their bones that old women move slower and time loses its immediacy. There is no point in rushing to get things done when waiting on the end.

I sat down for a visit with an old woman the other day. She listened politely as I shared news and told stories of trial and triumph. She nodded, sipped her tea, nibbled on a piece of pie. When all my words were spoken, she put on her apron and said, "It's time to get the dishes done."

The old woman knows the joys and sorrows of life

come and go, but the dishes always need to be done. Dishes, daily chores, provide a touch stone to the chaos of the day. She knows it is the familiar motions moved through every day with tedium that are the containers of our lives, that save us from the overwhelming and unknown world.

From one point of view Saturn was once the edge of the known Universe and Cailleach was the old woman who gives us enduring landmarks in the wilderness: a language for the unfamiliar offering us familiarity. From another point of view Saturn and Cailleach offer a chance to ask, what is beyond the familiar? Beyond meaning? Beyond the known?

Saturn and Cailleach provide us with limits that ask: is a stone more than just a stone, the darkness contained in the night sky more than just darkness and are we more than we suspect? These old ones ask, what are your limits? Or more importantly, what is on the other side?

Imagine you are standing in your garden. It is a nice day, not too hot, and not too cold. The cosmos' blooms are swaying in a breeze and a bee is buzzing. Your garden is familiar. Looking around you notice weeds you need to dig out and you admire how nicely you painted the table you found at the garage sale. Now look beyond the familiar, beyond your flowers, the weeds and table. Feel the unfamiliar woven through the familiar. Open to the chaos edging its way over your fences, up the walk and onto the back step. Consider for a moment the creative swirling life veiled by the familiar. Feel the presence of the weed beyond its intrusion into your sense of order. Sense the timelessness of the language shared by the bee and the flower.

Sometimes it's hard to feel the weaving between the cosmos flower and bee, the weed and the soil and your place in the garden beyond being the puller of weeds and the planter of flowers. For some people, the familiar is a veil that blurs their sense of place, their sense of belonging, in life. The veil deafens the call of the rose beckoning delight in the softness of its petal, or numbs the wonder of the timeless swirl on sunflower's face, or dulls the feeling of being embraced by the presence of place. The veil of certainty, words with singular meanings and the hard edges of limits, for some create a story that no longer is a story, but a singular reality.

We all know veils can be lifted. There are special plants that do this. Plants ruled by Saturn know how to lift the veil. Belladonna is one such plant. Belladonna's botanical name is Atropa belladonna. The plant is named after the ancient Greek Goddess Atropos. Atropos is the oldest Greek Goddess of Fate. She carries the scissors that cut the thread of life. Belladonna is a plant that lifts the greatest veil of all, the thin breath between life and death.

Belladonna's unusual medicine has not made this wayside weed popular.

In 1597, English herbalist John Gerard, a man who cultivated relationships with the rich and powerful of the English Court, in his herbal *Generall Historie of Plantes* described Belladonna as a "vile and filthy plant... long and lustful...wicked femme fatal, dark lady or whore." He advised, "eradication (of Belladonna) from a civilized place is the way to control the evil threat." (Gerard, 1663).

I think Dr Gerard was a wee bit hysterical.

Gerard's hatred of Belladonna probably wasn't caused by the plant's ability to cause death if taken in large amounts. Its ability to numb the body and shut down consciousness was used by ancient Greeks during surgeries and is still in use today. Gerard, a surgeon before becoming an herbalist, would have been trained to use Belladonna for surgeries. Having a patient unconscious while cutting into their flesh makes the life of a surgeon easier.

Gerard's hatred of Belladonna was more than likely due to its association with witches. Belladonna was a common ingredient in the old-time remedies called Flying Ointments, the ointment that was believed to give witches the gift of flight. At the time of publishing his herbal, persecution of witches by fire was erupting in towns and villages throughout Europe. Gerard would have wanted to distance himself from the women who used Belladonna to ease pain - physical, mental and spiritual.

In 1525 Bartolommeo Spina, a Dominican Inquisitor in Northern Italy, recorded this story about a young woman's persecution after using a Flying Ointment containing Belladonna.

He wrote of a young medical student who after a night at the ale house, discovered he had misplaced his key. He banged on the door to his lodgings and no one answered. He climbed up onto a balcony and entered the house through a window. He then went in search of the maid servant. When he entered her room, he found her unconscious on the floor, looking like death. He felt for her pulse. It was weak but steady. So, he left the girl there.

In the morning the medical student asked the maid about what had happened to her the night before. She replied that she'd been on a journey. The man reported this story to Bartolommeo the Inquisitor and the woman was arrested, tried and set on fire.

I can imagine the extreme limitations of the young maid's life. Not only was she responsible for cleaning up after a house full of young male students and feeding them, but this particular student also felt comfortable entering her room, drunk in the middle of the night.

Belladonna and the Flying Ointment must have been a balm of freedom for her weary spirit, silenced mind and exhausted body. Belladonna took her beyond the limitations of a poor serving girl subject to the whims and desires of those who considered themselves her betters. Belladonna, a magic plant, released her freedom-loving spirit trapped in a weighty world that limited her movement, speech and autonomy of her body.

Belladonna, a plant ruled by Saturn, unveils the paradox of limits. There is always the limitlessness on the other side of limits.

Flying Ointment has been known for a very long time. In the ancient Greek story, the Golden Ass of Asclepius, Pamphile, the first woman to spin silk and use the distaff to twist a thread from cotton wool, and not surprisingly called the Witch on the Isle of Thessaly, used a similar ointment.

> First Pamphile took off all her clothes. Then she opened a box and removed several small jars from it. She took the lid off one of these and scooped out some ointment, which she massaged for some time between her palms and then smeared it all over her body from the tips of her toenails to the top of her hair. After a long secret conversation with her lamp she began to shake her limbs in a quivering tremor. While her body undulated smoothly, soft down sprouted through her skin, and strong wing-feathers grew out; her nose hardened and curved, and her toenails bent into hooks. Pamphile had become an owl. (Muller-Ebeling, et al., 1998).

I BEGAN GROWING BELLADONNA A FEW YEARS AGO. IT is a gangly plant and a bit weedy but has a seductiveness to it. Belladonna's allure is not like the rose's beauty and perfume, but more like a woman behind a veil. Eventually you really want to see her true face. The veil keeps taunting you, "Take a peek." Eventually I had to try its infamous medicine.

First, I asked around to see what others had done, as I am well aware that Belladonna can be deadly. I am not particularly interested in the hallucinatory experiences Belladonna is famous for, nor did I want to collapse on the floor with a faint pulse as the maid did.

Belladonna at higher doses shuts down the sympathetic nervous system to the point where both breathing and the heart stops resulting in death. I definitely did not want to take my experimentation to this point. I just wanted to lift the veil.

So carefully considering my options in using Belladonna, I eventually decided to make a flower essence. A flower essence is what herbalists call energetic medicine. A very small amount of a plant's medicinal constituents are extracted in the process of making flower essence. This tiny amount of plant medicine gently nudges and opens the emotional body woven through flesh and bone and unravels tangled beliefs that contribute to ill health.

On a sunny morning, in early August, I picked Belladonna's flowers, dusky purple and bell-shaped, and placed them in a crystal bowl with fresh spring water. The water and the flowers mingled with sunlight all morning. Then I diluted the water down with brandy to preserve the medicine.

Since then, I have taken Belladonna many times. I have shared it with many friends, particularly my friends with a fondness for all things green. I have never taken enough to lay myself flat out on the floor and journey to wondrous lands.

When my friends and I have taken four drops of this special medicine, the veil between worlds is lifted and the unfamiliar sparkles through the familiar. A few drops of Belladonna and stones, plants, animals, other humans, glisten with something beyond the ordinary and everything becomes simple and free as the world gently hums it singular love song.

It is not surprising Belladonna is a maligned plant. Walking through life graced with knowing life's love song and seeing the great mystery woven through everyday tedium, you become a little wild. It is hard to be a good consumer when everything you could want is already present. It is hard to believe heaven could be anywhere else.

Besides the sparkle Belladonna brings to life, the plant opens us to threads of connection between life. Belladonna shows us how we are threaded into life's weaving. Belladonna renews our relationship with life and all its wilderness. The thread Belladonna stitches life back together with is a love song singing of the beauty found in the unfamiliar. Belladonna unveils Nature and all her wonder.

Like Belladonna, Cailleach with her standing stones and sacred wells, also weaves us into relationship with life's wilderness. Cailleach gives us the language of landmarks to understand our place among the mountains and whirlpools, both inner and outer. Cailleach allows the unfamiliar to weave itself into the familiar with respect and dignity.

Cailleach did not fare well when the Church planted its seed in the islands in the North Sea. While other ancient goddesses were given the honorific of Saint and took the veil of the nuns, the Cailleach, the Veil, the one who sparkles through the familiar, the hidden language of Nature, was dismissed as old women's tales.

As time passed, children were told baneful stories about the Cailleach. Beliefs were planted in their mind not to trust the Cailleach's ways.

Not so long ago, when the Cailleach scolded a boy who was shaking out the hay when rain was imminent, he challenged her, "How do you know it is going to rain, Old Woman?"

The Cailleach began to teach the boy the language of nature, "Because the scald-crow screamed it and the deer spoke it."

The boy scoffed and responded, "Heed not the scald-crow or the deer and heed not a woman's words. Whether it's early or later the sun rises. The day will be as God wills."

And so, a veil fell over the boy's eyes. Nature was no longer alive for him. The unfamiliar mingling with the familiar faded, unseen, unheard.

Sadly, today many people are frightened by wild places, the wind and dark nights. A veil of beliefs about singular existence and nature's non-livingness has set limits on the human story. Our containers are small with the unknown excluded. We are taught that the chaos of wild places must be controlled. We have lost our ability to see beyond the names of things and to live in the presence of place. The human being's value is measured in seconds, minutes and hours.

Not believing that mountains breathe the essence of life, nor forests, nor lakes, has allowed greed to overtake the human heart.

Limited definitions of life unleash greed. Cailleach's touch gave humans an upright stance that allows us to see in the distance. When humans are boxed in and cannot look beyond the walls of limited beliefs, a quiet voice always asks, is there is more? When divorced and fearful of Nature's wilderness and wonder, that small voice becomes greed. It's always a choice, do limits become limitless greed or limitless wonder.

Choose limitless greed and Cailleach hears the dog bark.

But wait a minute, there are still the plants like Belladonna that mingle the familiar with the unfamiliar. A few drops and stones begin to sing, trees sparkle and flowers sigh. It's a plant that opens eyes and ears to see and hear the livingness of the web. Saturn teaches us to look beyond the veil, discard the limits of belief and tell another ending. What are the limits of life? The limits of love? Plants like Belladonna bring us back to life. Feel the intimacy of place. Consider the edges of your story. Listen, do you hear the Cailleach's voice in the wind?

SATURN, BONES, AND COMFREY

The heat arrived early this morning. The pines are releasing their sharp, clean scent. The warm air carries the pine's scented molecules into the sky where they begin to seed clouds. I climb the hill slowly, saving my strength for the steeper climb up ahead. The back of my neck feels sweaty. I would welcome an afternoon rain. Lily, my eighty-five-pound dog, loops through the pines following her nose. She is following the scent of bones.

The first spring I walked in this forest, Lily brought me a deer's femur with thin scraps of periosteum, the transparent tissue that wraps bones, dangling from it like an Oak leaf in winter. Winter's deep snow had slowed the deer's movement until exhausted, she had lain down. The snow continued to fall. Holding the long thin bone, I feel the deer's final breath, a wisp of warm air in a cold night.

During the summer, Lily had shown me a squirrel's vertebrae threaded together with bits of ligament and torn red flesh. I wondered why the coyote had abandoned its meal. In the late fall, after the leaves had dropped, Lily led me to a moose skull and fear shivered through my body. The skull had been severed from its body by a sharp blow. Tender red stumps protruded from the skull where the antlers had been cleaved from bone. Flecks of earth-coloured skin clung to its great jaws. Its empty eye socket stared at me. Gruesome images of moose's last moments flashed through my mind.

Finding bones in the forest always wakes me to the moment. There is something about found bones that sends tremors deep into my soul like a greeting and a warning. Unearthed bones intrigue me. I feel their sacredness wrapped in the potency of silence. I want to touch them and step away at the same time. I feel the need to both cover them with dirt and leaves and tuck them into my backpack and slip away with them. Bones ruled by Saturn contain the hidden truths we either choose to unearth or leave buried.

From Iceland to India there are folk tales about truth telling bones. In each tale, there is a murder and a hastily dug grave. The murderer lies about the bloody deed. Eventually the family no longer seeks the lost one. Then, years later, when the missing one is almost forgotten, a finger bone pokes up from a muddy riverbank or a dog digs up a rib.

The strange part of these stories is the bones are usually discovered by a shepherd. He whittles away at the found bone to make a flute. When the shepherd plays his new flute, the instrument sings a terrible tale of murder. The perpetuator is discovered and tried. Saturn's hard cold truth prevails.

The bones of Richard III, King of England from 1483 to 1485, were found under a parking lot in Leicester, England in 2012. They had lain in the earth, bony wrist folded as if bound, for 527 years.

Shakespeare, hired by the Queen of England whose grandfather had played a role in the murder of Richard III, wrote a play of Richard's life. In Shakespeare's play Richard III is a Machiavellian tyrant who murders children, his nephews, to seize the throne. The story goes that because Richard is ugly and a hunchback he is embittered by his misfortune. He ruthlessly covets what others of a gentler appearance are given. Shakespeare portrays Richard's death as a great boon for England.

The discovery of Richard's bones exposed the brutality of his murder. After 500 years in a shallow grave, Richard's bones revealed he was attacked by someone carrying a sword and suffered several head wounds and blows to ribs. Perhaps the same person, or another, plunged a dagger into Richard's head leaving a penetrating wound at the top of his skull. The final catastrophic blow was caused by a halberd, a razor-sharp axe blade attached to a long pole, that almost severed his head from his body. After death his pelvic bone revealed one final humiliating wound. His corpse had been stabbed in the buttocks with a dagger.

Richard's bones not only brought to light the horror of his death, but also created interest in the truth of his character buried in the libellous propaganda spread by his murderers. Richard is now portrayed as a generous, thoughtful and fair ruler. He did not have a hunchback but was disfigured by sever sclerosis. He is described as being stoic in the face of the pain his crooked spine would have caused. Whether or not he ordered the assassination of his brother's children is a matter of debate. Many believe it was his murderers who took the lives of his nephews. Richard III was not the man Queen Elizabeth I, granddaughter of the man who led the rebellion against Richard, portrayed him to be.

Elizabeth was the first English monarch to take an interest in the New World. In 1578, Elizabeth sent Humphrey Gilbert to explore and colonize territories unclaimed by Christian kingdoms. And so, the trail of bones across Canada, left behind by colonization, began, my Great-Great-Grandmother Elsie's bones amongst them.

I imagine Elsie, uprooted from Scotland, emerging from the dark hull of the ship as she squints in the bright sunlight. It is dizzying, stepping from the ship that had carried her and her children across the stormy Atlantic and onto firm ground. She is weak with hunger. Her youngest, sick with fever clings to her soiled skirts. She has not changed her clothes once in six weeks of the voyage.

Her eldest, jaw set, bravely hauls their heavy trunk. Elsie's heart skips a beat when she loses sight of her middle boy in the crowd. With two of her children, Elsie is funnelled towards the men recording names and dates in ledgers. She desperately scans the crowd for her boy's blond hair. She spies him up ahead in the line with the friend he'd made on the crossing.

Elsie feels in her pocket for the carefully wrapped seeds. They are her good luck charm during this difficult time. She had collected the seeds from her garden at home: St. John's Wort, Angelica, Nettle, Violet and Valerian. In the chaos of unwashed, malnourished bodies seeking a new life, she imagines her garden of healing plants. Elsie will grow her plants to mend and knit her family back together.

From one packet of seeds, she will grow a plant commonly called Comfrey, a plant ruled by Saturn. When she was a girl her mother had taught her the plant's name was Knitbone. Her mother also showed her how to make a cast with its leaves to heal broken bones and poultices to repair torn skin. Today, any herbalist with an herb garden has a patch of comfrey. It is one of the first herbs herbalist learn about in school.

I taught for a little while at an herbal school in Toronto. Once when I was prepared to teach a weekend course on herbal medicine and cancer, I was suddenly asked to share what I know about the Doctrine of Signatures. Confused by the abrupt change in plans and completely unprepared to teach The Doctrine of Signatures, the ancient art of understanding a plant's medicine through careful examination of its appearance, scent, taste and the environment where it grows, I said, "Okay," and hoped for the best.

The school was in a downtown neighbourhood, densely packed with people. The entire area was either cemented over or covered in hard compact soil trod on day and night. The noise of cars and sirens was irritating, and the air was infused with the smell of garbage mingled with exhaust fumes.

The only plants growing near the school are straggly weeds emerging from the cracks in pavement and the narrow fissures between the building's foundation and the street. I was feeling a little overwhelmed by the thought of sitting in a back alley amongst the cigarette butts and stench of urine meditating on a sprig of Shepard's Purse seeking light in the shadow of a dumpster. Then, miraculously someone arrived with a bucket of Comfrey roots, dirt still clinging to their smooth black skin.

The students knew Comfrey had once been called Knitbone. They also knew it contains a phytoconstituent, allantoin, that encourages healing of broken tissue. We were off to a good start.

The students carefully peeled back the smooth black skin to expose the bone white fleshy roots. Comfrey's white, thick roots are a clear signature that the plant carries medicine for bones. Then the magic happened.

Sometimes, when we open up to plants and ask them to teach us their medicine, time shifts, perception alters, and a potent silence engulfs hearts and minds. It is like an overarching presence that understands the mystery of life, both human and plant, descends weaving roots with hands, eyes with leaf and hearts with the plant's essence. For a short time, human and plant are intertwined in deep communion. It is a spaciousness that fosters understanding between two distinct intelligences, human and plant, interconnected since before time was remembered. A direct, wise and undeniable knowing takes place between people and plants without words but with feelings.

When communication with plants happens in this way it is like an ancient spell has been cast, altering senses, opening intuition, and an understanding of the plant's spirit is unveiled. This is what happened that day in the downtown classroom. Everyone in the class felt it.

Suddenly we were no longer speaking of healing bones and phytoconstituents. We were giving voice to a plant that understands buried bones. We spoke about ancestors and memories held in bones. We realized that Comfrey does not just heal bones—it knows bones.

Last summer, Lily dug up a midden, a refuse heap, in the back corner of my garden. I had moved a shed that had been there for years. Under it was buried rusted tin cans, old medicine bottles, a clock with its hands stuck at 3:35 and bones. I laid out the bones and objects in front of me and tried to image who had buried them there. I asked my neighbour what she thought.

"We all buried our trash out back in the day," was all she said.

The bones resembled the cow bones I bring home for Lily from the butcher. In the fall, I dug up a part of my garden to bury them again. Bones are good for the garden. They offer nutrients to both the plants and the mycelium. Comfrey does this too.

The Comfrey seeds Elsie carried in her pocket were not only to grow plants for casts and poultices, but also to nourish her garden's soil. Today, after an herbalist makes her oils and teas with Comfrey's roots and leaves, she chops up the rest to add to her compost to feed next year's plants.

Comfrey, while helpful, can quickly become a menace in the garden if not restrained. It carries Saturn's dominating influence. If unchecked, Comfrey will overwhelm a garden suffocating and choking out the more delicate plants in its path.

In the garden, Comfrey must be planted in the place where it will remain. If Comfrey is moved, from each broken root another plant will spring. Once Comfrey takes root, it is almost impossible to eradicate. If left to its own devices the garden becomes a hostile patch of prickly leaves (Comfrey has prickly leaves) and stubborn, deeply penetrating roots.

Infused with Saturn's energy Comfrey will either feed the garden or destroy it. Saturn will nourish you with respect or crush you with dominance. It's your choice.

When Elsie joined her husband at the homestead just outside of Guelph, Ontario, I wonder what she did with the native plants that were already there. The maple forest would have been abundant with Blue Cohosh, Goldenseal, False Unicorn Root, American Ginseng, all endangered medicinal plants now. I image generations of these plants enjoying the shade of the great maples that Elsie and those who arrived with her were quickly hewing down and turning into homes, barns, wagons and furniture. Not understanding the community of life these plants belonged to or the medicine they carried, did she dig them out and replace them with the seeds from her pocket?

It was like that when the settlers arrived in North America. They were searching for a home like the one they left behind. They did not know the name of the strange forest plants with their delicate flowers and deep roots. The forest's dark shadows and animals long extinct in the lands they came from were threatening. They did not understand the forest's silent language of mycelium and roots, scents and clouds, medicine and the human body. Seeking some simple familiarity amongst the wild strangeness, Elsie planted Comfrey and Angelica, Nettles and Mugwort. Like Comfrey uprooted in the garden, the plants spread taking up the spaces where native species grew.

Just as Elsie did not recognize the plants that grew in her forested homestead, the people who lived in the great forests were difficult for her to understand. She did not know these brown-skinned people understood the silent language of the forest. Their dark brown, almost black eyes shone with a stillness that disturbed Elsie's industriousness. Their language that sounded like running water and wind in trees was gibberish to her ears. Their belief that nature was alive flew in the face of her Christian conviction that "man has dominion over nature." Elsie was shrouded by the protestant work ethic: diligence, discipline and frugality bring to life God's grace. This is a creed infused by Saturn's most rigid vibration, austerity, a way of life that denies other beliefs. Denial—another of Saturn's challenges.

If there was a planetary rulership assigned to colonization, I would suggest Saturn. The incredibly hard work of early Europeans who "built this country" carries Saturn's vibration of earnest diligence and sacrifice. Yet this country is also built on the hidden truth of the many bones lying in hastily dug graves. It is a truth that cuts close to bone in defiance of the story many still cling to—a land that is strong and free.

Terry Glavin, in his article Truth and Native Abuse writes:

> Indian country, as we used to call it, is a vast landscape of tombs. And the dead are still there, among and between the houses of reborn, thriving villages, and among and between the crumbling ruins of mission chapels, church-run tuberculosis hospitals, dormitories, and residential schools.After all this suffering, the very least we owe the dead, and the living, is the truth. (Glavin, 2008).

THERE ARE HASTILY DUG GRAVES ALONG THE TRAIL OF Tears that crisscross this country. These trails mark the enforced marches of Indigenous people from traditional lands to foreign reservations.

There are hastily dug graves of Indigenous families overcome by rashes and fever.

There are shallow graves of Indigenous children behind abandoned buildings with broken windows once call schools.

There are the graves of missing and murdered Indigenous women. Some say as many as 1200 since

1969 have gone missing. Many have been found murdered. Since Elsie's time, no one knows the number of Indigenous women buried—somewhere.

I had the privilege of sitting in a series of circles over a long winter with a group of Indigenous and Metis women and men endeavouring to heal the deep cuts in their souls made by the loss of a daughter, cousin, aunt, sister, mother, wife. These women had disappeared one day and were never seen again—unless their bones were found in a ditch, off a mining road, deep in the forest or in a pig's pen.

Being a white woman and having ancestors who turned their eyes away from the grinding poverty of reservations and the abuse in residential schools, I rarely spoke in the circles. I learned to listen deeply.

Within the circles silence hoovered between words, tears and laughter. The silence held the stories in a gentle embrace and welcomed the pain and the love present. The circles were deeply moving and disturbed core beliefs about justice, fairness, truth and lies.

The women who are missing and murdered are not just drunks and prostitutes, but people with families and friends, joys and sorrows. Many are teenagers naive enough to take a ride with a stranger.

In the circle, listening with care and gentleness, the bones of women in hastily dug graves could be heard. There was a sacred presence in the circles that dove deeply into the heart of a person willing to hear and allow space for stories untold. The silence woven into the sorrow, anger and bitterness transcended words and led to the understanding of the heart.

It takes Saturn's steely eye to gaze upon the truth of bones in hastily dug graves. We are living in a time when to turn away, to put on Saturn's cloak of denial, "We were only trying to survive," is no longer acceptable. It's time to listen for the silence of the stories not told.

To one of the circles special guests were invited. They were a white family whose daughter went missing along what is called The Highway of Tears. The highway is also called The Yellowhead and runs from Winnipeg, through Edmonton and all the way to the British Columbia Coast.

As the highway winds through central BC between Prince George and Prince Rupert it links First Nations communities, logging and mining camps and small towns where services like doctors, grocery stores and banks are found. There are miles and miles of highway surrounded by wilderness. Along this stretch of highway, since 1970, it is estimated 40 women have gone missing. From 1989 to 2006 nine young women went missing or were found murdered in the woods along the highway. All the women but one was Indigenous.

The one white woman, a tree planter who disappeared without a trace was the daughter of the special guests in the circle. They had been invited because the Native Elders in the community did not want to shut out the pain of their loss. They wanted to open to the pain of the white girls' parents to allow it become part of the whole, the whole which includes hundreds of other women murdered and missing.

The silence was penetrating and still in the circle that day. Sometimes truth can only be told with silence.

The land my ancestors cleared will never again be vast forests, crystal clear waters and plains dotted with Echinacea and roamed by buffalo. Many people are working towards rebuilding populations of Blue Cohosh, Goldenseal, American Ginseng, False Unicorn. Yet, we cannot bring back the dead. Often, we can't even find their bones.

But we can no longer say, "I didn't know."

Today cities brighten night's darkness and highways stretching for miles and miles. Anything is possible with the push of a button. Arctic ice melts, forests burn, and soil is poisoned. At this precious time in history there is a great cry for change, a change that requires discipline and sacrifice, both qualities Saturn offers. It is time to limit uncontained growth and nourish the container of life. It is time to find the discipline necessary to discover the meaning within the centre of our being, not in that which lies outside our skin. It is time to recognize that no matter where we stand, under our feet the bones of ancestors lie.

Comfrey with its Saturnine qualities can show us how to move forward from the devastation of the past. Comfrey heals broken bones and torn skin by bringing in new life. It speeds the development of new cells to replace those that were injured. Comfrey makes wounds whole again by weaving in health.

Saturn brings the jaw dropping, sinking feeling of the moment when you realize you were wrong. Saturn blindsides you. It shows you the truth of choices made. Then Saturn leaves it up to you to decide how to move forward—pretend you did not notice Saturn's entrance into your life, or seek the new understanding.

Healing is not returning to what was. It is moving onto the new.

Once the truth has been told, heard, understood and embodied, the healing is complete. Walk away and don't look back. Picking at scabs only prolongs the pain. Saturn rips off the band-aid to reveal the mended tissue.

Sitting in the circle with my Indigenous friends, listening to generations of pain and injustice, feeling them welcome a white woman who had lost her daughter, just as they had lost their sisters, mothers, daughters, and afterwards sitting around drinking coffee and eating donuts, laughing as a comic three-year-old showed us her dance moves, taught me the sacred discipline of silence and healing of shared joy.

And those bones, the one's buried in shallow graves? When it is time they will rise to the surface. Their story will be told. Saturn can't turn a blind eye forever. Eventually the truth will be told.

For More:

Abrah offers workshops and webinars on herbal medicine, healing and a three year apprenticeship program in Clinical Herbalism. Abrah is available for individual health consultations and speaking engagements.

. . .

Abrah's previously published books are The Herbal Apprentice: Plant Medicine and the Human Body.

https://www.amazon.ca/s?k=Abrah+Arneson+the+Herbal+Apprentice&i=stripbooks&ref=nb_sb_noss

Its accompanying workbook is called The Herbal Apprentice Workbook. Both books can be found on Amazon.

Currently Abrah is working on a new book, Herbal Medicine: Bacteria, Viruses and Parasites.

For more information about Abrah's offerings, writings and service please go to her website: www.abraherbs.com

WORKS CITED

Apuleius, & Walsh, P. G. (1994). *The Golden Ass*. Oxford: Clarendon Press.

Bacon, Francis. Spedding, James (Ed.), Ellis, Robert Leslie (Eds.) Heath, Douglas Denon (Eds.). (1857-1874). Vol 6. *The Works of Francis Bacon: The Wisdom of the Ancients.* P.747. Cambridge, England. Cambridge University Press.

———Novum Organum, 1620

———Ibid.

———"Advancement of Learning," in The Great Books: Advancement of Learning, Novum Organum, New Atlantis, The Great Books of the Western World (n.p.: Encyclopædia Britannica, 1980).

Baconnier Simon, Lang Sydney B., de Seze Rene. (2002). "*New Crystal in the Pineal Gland: characterization and potential role in electromechano transduction.*" *27. URSI General*

Assembly, Aug 2002, Maastricht, Netherlands. ⟨ineris-00972373⟩

Bartram, Dr. Thomas. (1998).*Bartram's Encyclopedia of Herbal Medicines.* Constable & Robinson.

Bennett, Judith, M. (1991). *Misogyny, Popular Culture and Women's Work* https://www.researchgate.net/publication/31120708_Misogyny_Popular_Culture_and_Women's_Work

Berke, Maggie Rose. (2017).*"Naturalized Women and Womanized Earth: Connecting the Journeys of Womanhood and the Earth, from the Early Modern Era to the Industrial Revolution". Senior Projects Spring 2017*. 290. https://digitalcommons.bard.edu/senproj_s2017/290

Brinton-Perera, Sylvia. (1981). *Descent to the Goddess.* Canada. Inner City Books.

Casini, E. (2018). *RETHINKING THE MULTIFACETED ASPECTS OF MANDRAKE IN ANCIENT EGYPT. Egitto E Vicino Oriente, 41*, 101-116. doi:10.2307/26774454

Cohen, Leonard. (1992.) *Anthem* on The Future.

Culpeper, Nicholas.(2019). *Culpeper's Complete Herbal & English Phys*. New York. Sterling.

Dashu Max. *Witches and Pagans: Women in European Folk Religion, 700-110*. Veleda Press, 2017.

Eurielle & Ryan Louder, 2017. *Midsummer's Song* on Goodbye Butterfly.

Euripides. (1925). *The Helen of Euripides.* Cambridge [Eng.] : The University Press.

Faulkes, Anthony. (Trans.) (1995: 28-29). Edda. *Everyman* https://en.wikipedia.org/wiki/Fenrir

Freeman Mara *Cauldron of Change* www.chalicecentre.net/cauldron-of-change.html 2021

Gerard, J., & In Johnson, T. (1636). *The Herball: Or generall historie of plantes.* London: Printed by A.I.J. Norton and R. Whitakers.

Glavin, Terry. *Truth and Native Abuse*. https://thetyee.ca/Views/2008/04/30/TruthAndAbuse/

Hall, Judy. (2003). *The Crystal Bible: A Definitive Guide to Crystals*. Walking Stick Press, Cincinnati, Ohio.

Homer. Fagles, R., & Knox, B. (1998). *The Iliad.*

Jones, Charlene. (1996). *Passion Seed.* Uncritical Mass in Consort. Sadhana Press, Toronto, Canada.

Jones, Mary http://www.maryjones.us/jce/towerhill.html

Kramer, Heinrich and Sprenger, Jacob. (1486). *Malleus Maleficarum*, Speyer, Germany.

LaBerge, Ph.D., Rheingold, Howard. (1991). *Exploring The World of Lucid Dreaming:* http://users.telenet.be/sterf/texts/other/exploring_the_world_of_lucid_dreaming.pdf Ballantine.

Mackenzie, D. M. (1917). *Wonder Tales from Scottish Myths and Legends.* Trieste Publishing Pty Ltd. The author is indebted for his description of Cailleach.

Mark, Joshua J. https://www.ancient.eu/article/215/inannas-descent-a-sumerian-tale-of-injustice/). 2011

Muller-Ebeling, C., Ratsch, Christian, Strol, Wolf-Deter, (2003) *Witchcraft Medicine: Healing Arts, Shamanic Practices and Forbidden Plants.* Inner Traditions, Rochester, Vermont.

Oates, Joyce Carol. (1990). *I Locked the Door Upon Myself.* Eco Press, New York.

Odenwold, Dr. Sten. (2003). (https://image.gsfc.nasa.gov/poetry/tour/AAmag.html#:~:text=The%20magnetic%20-field%20of%20Earth,the%20crust%20and%20enters%20space.)

Oren, Dr. Sarah. (https://pubmed.ncbi.nlm.nih.gov/2062202/)

Persinger,Michael. (2001). https://neuro.psychiatryonline.org/doi/full/10.1176/jnp.13.4.515

Ronder, Tanya, Levin, Hanoch, Euripides. The Shed, London England (2013). *The Lost Women of Troy* by Hanoch Levin, working adaptation by Tanya Ronder.

Sjoo and Moore. (1987). *The Great Cosmic Mother: Rediscovering the Religion of the Earth.* Harper Collins, San Francisco.

Wynn, E.S. *Sky Wolves Lost Constellations and Stellar Magic in Old Norse and Ancient European Cosmology* (2020). Lulu.com

For the stories of Airmed and Miach and the Old Woman and Bones the author is indebted to https://cailleachs-herbarium.com/2015/08/the-cailleach-a-tale-of-balance-between-darkness-and-light-part-two/

For the tale of Taliesin the author is indebted to https://www.bbc.co.uk/wales/history/sites/themes/society/myths_taliesin.shtml

ACKNOWLEDGMENTS

The seed for The Weaving was planted by the beautiful, loving and funny Teresa Corky Larson Jonasson. I am so grateful for her presence in my life. Tiffany Freeman watered the seed with her generous sharing. Thank you, Tiffany for your courage to stand with a foot in both worlds.

Over many years there have been many conversations that nourished The Weaving. I wish to thank Beige MacIntosh, Megan Spenser and Marianne Beacon for sharing your insights over tea at my kitchen table. Dionne Jennings and Penny Beaudrow, thank you for always being there on the other end of the phone. Lunch with Hanna Williams has fed me with encouragement for The Weaving on many afternoons between clients.

Thank you to all those who participated in the Ancestor Story Webinars throughout COVID and kindly offered me your encouragement to keep writing, in particular Kimmy and DC Michaels who always showed up. My heart bursts with gratitude to Charlene Jones who guided me through the last hurdles of The Weaving with wisdom and kindness. She makes my writing so much better.

I could not have written this book without Mark Arneson. He patiently navigated piles of books on every flat surface in our house for months. He spent hours answering questions about planets and poking holes in my endless theories about astrology. He gave me space when I needed it and was always ready to read, listen and advise.

I need to thank the Plants. They have enriched my life in ways that I could have never imagined. I am grateful to the light the Planets shine in the night sky. They continue to inspire me.

And to the Storytellers, thank you for remembering. Lastly, to my Grandmothers who just want me to be happy, Vera Kirkman and Elsie Newton, thank you.

ABOUT THE AUTHOR

Most people have an essential question in their life. This question is their beacon. Some would even say this question is their karma. Abrah's question is: how can life's intoxicating beauty co-exist with the depth of despair and suffering life can bring?

This question led Abrah to work in hospice supporting the dying, train as a doula to hold women while they laboured, travel to all continents on this planet and spend a year in retreat in the Yukon wilderness.

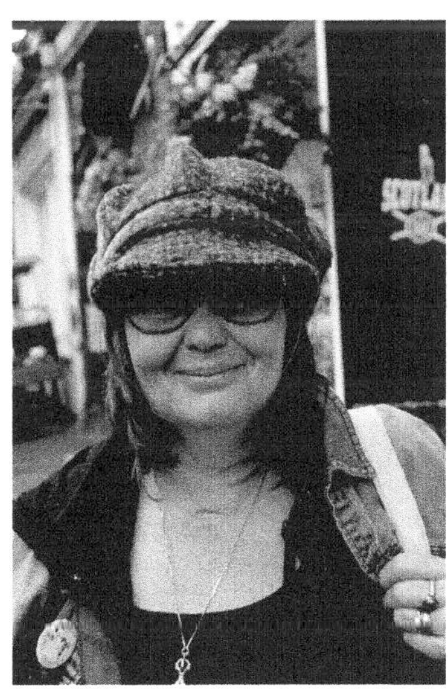

She has been practicing Clinical Herbal Medicine for almost 20 years, has nourished this question and deepened her understanding of transformation from illness to health, from despair to hope and from disconnection to connection.

Abrah is the author of *The Herbal Apprentice: Plant Medicine and The Human Being* and *The Herbal Apprentice Workbook.*

Currently she practices herbal medicine in Ottawa, Ontario and leads a herbal apprentice program in the Gatineau in Quebec.

Find her at www.abraherbs.com or facebook at Abrah Herbalist in the Woods

ALSO BY ABRAH ARNESON

For More:

Abrah offers workshops and webinars on herbal medicine, healing and a three year apprenticeship program in Clinical Herbalism. Abrah is available for individual health consultations and speaking engagements.

Abrah's previously published books are The Herbal Apprentice: Plant Medicine and the Human Body.

www.amazon.ca/Herbal-Apprentice-Plant-Medicine
Human/dp/0993906907/ref=sr_1_1?
dchild=1&keywords=abrah+arneson&qid=1615903291&sr=8-1

Its accompanying workbook is called The Herbal Apprentice Workbook. Both books can be found on Amazon.

www.amazon.ca/Herbal-Apprentice-Work
Book/dp/0993906923/ref=sr_1_2?
dchild=1&keywords=abrah+arneson&qid=1615903342&sr=8-2

Currently Abrah is working on a new book, Herbal Medicine: Bacteria, Viruses and Parasites.

For more information about Abrah's offerings, writings and service please go to her website: www.abraherbs.com

Made in the USA
Monee, IL
16 June 2021

71504510R00148